TB Essentials: A Pocket Guide Demystifying Diagnosis

Reviewed & Foreword by

Kakithakara Vajravelu Leela

Professor and Head – Microbiology & Associate Dean (UG Studies)
SRM MCH & RC, SRMIST

Author

Sujith Sri Surya Ravi

Assistant Professor - Microbiology, SRM MCH & RC, SRMIST

Co-Author & Editor

Maheswary Datchanamoorthy

Associate Professor - Microbiology, SRM MCH & RC, SRMIST

First Edition
March 2025

TB Essentials: A Pocket Guide Demystifying Diagnosis

Foreword & Reviewer: *Kakithakara Vajravelu Leela*

Author and Self Publisher: *Sujith Sri Surya Ravi*

Co-Author & Editor: *Maheswary Datchanamoorthy*

Edition: First Edition (21st March 2025)

Self-Published under the banner of Institution
SRM Institute of Science and Technology (Deemed to be University u/s 3 of UGC Act 1956) - Formerly known as SRM University

Publishing Address / Author's Correspondence details
Sujith Sri Surya R, Department of Microbiology, SRM Medical College Hospital and Research Centre, Faculty of Medicine and Health Sciences, SRM Institute of Science and Technology, SRM Nagar, Kattankulthur, Chengalpattu District, Tamilnadu - 603203, India. Mobile – 9791101782 / 9176355673, Mail ID – sujithsrisurya@gmail.com

ISBN: 978-93-342-5841-7 for E-Book (Kindle) and Paperback Imprinting

ISBN: 979-83-160-5087-1 for Amazon Hardcover Copies Imprinting

Cover pages Design and Typeset are self-worked.

Published in India, for print and electronic reading worldwide.

Disclaimer
The information presented in this book is for educational and reference purposes only. While every effort has been made to ensure accuracy, the author(s) and publisher are not responsible for any errors or omissions, or for any outcomes resulting from the use of this information. Readers are advised to consult medical professionals or official guidelines for clinical decision-making. Medical knowledge is constantly changing. As new information becomes available, changes in treatment, procedure, equipment and use of drugs becomes necessary. Please consult full prescribing information before issuing prescriptions for any product mentioned in this publication.

Foreword

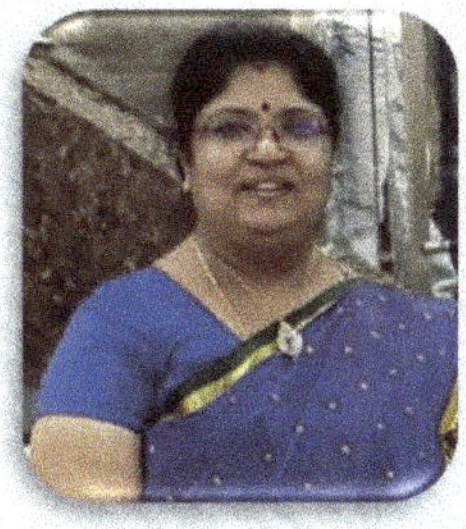

Prof. Dr. K. V. Leela *M.D.(Micro) D.G.O.,*
Head of Microbiology Department & Associate Dean (UG Studies)
SRM Medical College Hospital and Research Centre,
Faculty of Medicine and Health Sciences,
SRM Institute of Science and Technology (SRM IST),
(Deemed to be University u/s 3 of UGC Act 1956)
Kattankulathur – 603203, Chengalpattu Dt., Tamilnadu, India.

Tuberculosis remains one of the most significant infectious diseases, posing a major public health challenge worldwide. Despite advances in diagnostics, treatment strategies, and global initiatives to combat TB, the disease continues to claim millions of lives each year. The need for comprehensive, accessible, and up-to-date knowledge on tuberculosis cannot be overstated, especially for medical professionals, researchers, and students who are at the forefront of this battle.

*It is with great pleasure that I introduce **TB Essentials: A Pocket Guide demystifying Diagnosis**, a well-structured and meticulously compiled resource that provides an in-depth understanding of tuberculosis, from its pathogenesis to the latest diagnostic and treatment modalities. This book is a testament to the dedication, expertise, and scholarly rigor of **Sujith Sri Surya R**, whose passion for tuberculosis research and commitment to medical education have culminated in this invaluable guide.*

*I extend my appreciation to **Dr. Maheswary Datchanamoorthy**, whose role as a co-author and reviewer has ensured the accuracy, clarity, and comprehensiveness of the content. Her meticulous approach to scientific detailing has significantly contributed to the quality of this book.*

This book not only serves as an academic reference but also as a practical guide for clinicians, microbiologists, and public health professionals engaged in the diagnosis and management of tuberculosis. By integrating fundamental concepts with the latest advancements in TB research, TB Essentials: A Pocket Guide demystifying Diagnosis stands as a crucial resource in bridging the gap between theory and practice.

I commend the authors and contributors for their tireless efforts in bringing this work to life. It is my sincere hope that this book will aid medical professionals in their pursuit of knowledge, enhance clinical decision-making, and ultimately contribute to the global effort to control and eliminate tuberculosis.

Kakithakara Vajravelu Leela
Reviewer of TB Essentials: A Pocket Guide demystifying Diagnosis

Author's Acknowledgment

Asst. Prof. SUJITH SRI SURYA R *M.Sc.(Med.Micro),PGDEAS,BAL,*
Department of Microbiology,
SRM Medical College Hospital and Research Centre,
Faculty of Medicine and Health Sciences,
SRM Institute of Science and Technology (SRM IST),
(Deemed to be University u/s 3 of UGC Act 1956)
Kattankulathur – 603203, Chengalpattu Dt., Tamilnadu, India.

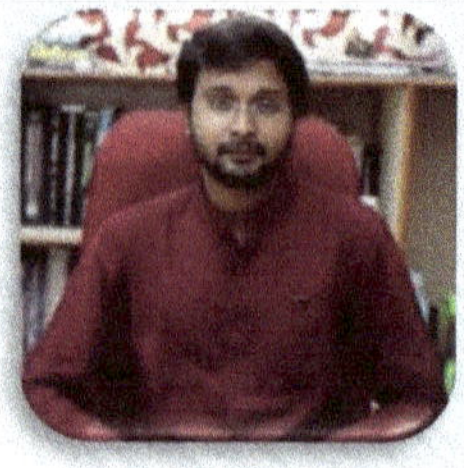

*The completion of this book, **TB Essentials: A Pocket Guide demystifying Diagnosis**, would not have been possible without the invaluable contributions of numerous individuals and my Institute. I express my heartfelt gratitude to all those who have supported and guided me throughout this endeavour.*

*First and foremost, I extend my sincere thanks to my mentors, **Head of Microbiology Department and Associate Dean (UG Studies) Prof. Dr. Kakithakara Vajravelu Leela**, a peer in the field of microbiology and tuberculosis research. Her dedication to academic and research excellence and commitment to maintaining the highest standards of scientific rigor have been truly commendable. Madam's critical review, insights, discussions, and encouragement have been instrumental in shaping the content of this book.*

*My sincere thanks go to Co-Author and Editor, **Dr. Maheswary Datchanamoorthy**, whose keen eye for detail and relentless efforts in refining the content meticulously have played a crucial role in ensuring the clarity and coherence of this book. And heartfelt appreciation to her as a dedicated editor, whose expertise in editing and structured approach in formatting the manuscript has been invaluable in bringing the final outline of the book.*

*A special thanks to **all my colleagues in the Department of Microbiology** for their unwavering support and for fostering an environment of academic excellence. A special note of gratitude to my family and friends for their unwavering patience and encouragement throughout this process. Their belief in my work has been a source of strength and perseverance.*

I would also like to acknowledge my students and research fellows, whose curiosity and dedication to learning have been a constant source of motivation. Their questions and discussions have enriched my perspective on tuberculosis diagnosis and treatment.

Finally, to all healthcare professionals, researchers, and policymakers dedicated to the fight against tuberculosis—this book is a tribute to your tireless efforts in combating this global health challenge. It is my hope that this guide serves as a useful resource in your mission to diagnose, treat, and ultimately eliminate TB.

Thank you all for being a part of this journey.

Sujith Sri Surya Ravi
Author of TB Essentials: A Pocket Guide demystifying Diagnosis

Co-Author and Editor's Acknowledgment

Assoc. Prof. Dr. D. Maheswary *M.D.(Micro),*
Department of Microbiology,
SRM Medical College Hospital and Research Centre,
Faculty of Medicine and Health Sciences,
SRM Institute of Science and Technology (SRM IST),
(Deemed to be University u/s 3 of UGC Act 1956)
Kattankulathur – 603203, Chengalpattu Dt., Tamilnadu, India.

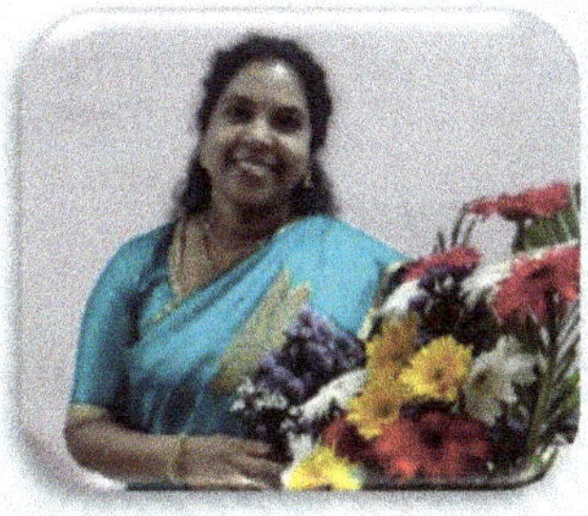

Being part of the creation of ***TB Essentials: A Pocket Guide demystifying Diagnosis*** *has been a rewarding experience, and we extend our heartfelt gratitude to those who have made this journey possible. This book is the result of collective efforts, and we acknowledge the contributions of many who have helped shape it into a valuable resource.*

I express my deepest gratitude to ***Prof. Dr. Kakithakara Vajravelu Leela****, Head of the Department of Microbiology and Associate Dean (UG Studies), for her constant encouragement, guidance, and unwavering support. Her invaluable insights have played a crucial role in refining the scientific content and ensuring the book's academic integrity.*

I thank ***Sujith Sri Surya Ravi****, the primary author, whose vision, expertise, and commitment to excellence have been the driving force behind this book. His passion for academics and research in diagnostic microbiology has been instrumental in ensuring the comprehensiveness and relevance of this guide.*

A special note of appreciation goes to the Department of Microbiology, SRM Medical College Hospital and Research Centre, for providing an inspiring environment that fosters research, collaboration, and academic excellence. The support of our colleagues has been invaluable throughout the development of this book.

We also recognize the contributions of students and research fellows whose curiosity, discussions, and engagement have enriched this work. Their enthusiasm for learning has motivated us to make this guide as informative and practical as possible.

Finally, this book is dedicated to all medical professionals, researchers, and policymakers who work tirelessly in the fight against tuberculosis. It is our hope that TB Essentials: A Pocket Guide demystifying Diagnosis serves as a valuable reference in advancing TB diagnosis, treatment, and prevention worldwide.

Thank you all for being a part of this endeavour.

Maheswary Datchanamoorthy
Co-Author & Editor of TB Essentials: A Pocket Guide demystifying Diagnosis

CONTENTS

- *WHO guidelines and diagnostic algorithms*

18. Sample Collection and Processing

- ***Pulmonary TB:*** *Sputum collection techniques (spot, morning, induced sputum)*
- ***Extrapulmonary TB:*** *Sample types (CSF, pleural fluid, gastric aspirates, FNAC, tissue biopsy, urine, blood)*
- ***Latent TB:*** *Blood and skin-based tests*
- *Sample transportation and biosafety considerations*

19. Microscopy-Based Diagnostics

- ***Ziehl-Neelsen (ZN) Staining***
    - *Principle, procedure, interpretation, limitations*
- ***Fluorescent Microscopy (Auramine-Rhodamine Staining)***
    - *Sensitivity comparison with ZN staining*
    - *Advantages in high-burden settings*
- ***LED Fluorescent Microscopy***
    - *WHO recommendations and field applications*
- ***Fluorescein Diacetate (Fda) Staining In Tuberculosis Diagnosis***
    - *Principle, Advantages, Clinical Applications and limitations*

20. *Culture-Based Diagnosis*

- ***Solid Culture Methods***
    - *Löwenstein-Jensen (LJ) Medium*
    - *Middlebrook 7H10 and 7H11 Media*
    - *Turnaround time and colony morphology interpretation*
- ***Liquid Culture Methods***
    - *Mycobacteria Growth Indicator Tube (MGIT)*
    - *BACTEC 460 Radiometric System*
    - *BACTEC 9000 MB and BacT/Alert MB Systems*
- ***Automated Culture Systems***
    - *Advantages in drug susceptibility testing (DST)*
    - *WHO recommendations on culture-based methods*

21. Molecular Diagnostics

- ***Nucleic Acid Amplification Tests (NAATs)***
    - ***GeneXpert MTB/RIF & GeneXpert Ultra***
        - *Principle, procedure, detection limits, interpretation*

        - *Rifampicin resistance detection and its clinical significance*
    - ***Line Probe Assay (LPA)***
        - *Genotypic DST for first-line and second-line drugs*
        - *Hain test (MTBDRplus, MTBDRsl) and newer advancements*
    - ***Loop-Mediated Isothermal Amplification (LAMP)***
        - *Advantages in resource-limited settings*
    - ***Whole-Genome Sequencing (WGS) and Next-Generation Sequencing (NGS)***
        - *Role in epidemiology, resistance prediction, and strain typing*
- ***Other PCR-Based Methods***
    - *Real-time PCR and conventional PCR techniques*
    - *Xpert XDR-TB: Detecting pre-XDR and XDR strains*

22. Immunodiagnostic Approaches

- ***Tuberculin Skin Test (TST, Mantoux Test)***
    - *Mechanism, interpretation, limitations*
    - *False positives/negatives and BCG interference*
- ***Interferon-Gamma Release Assays (IGRAs)***
    - *QuantiFERON-TB Gold Plus*
    - *T-SPOT.TB test*
    - *Comparative sensitivity and specificity*
    - *Applications in latent TB infection (LTBI) diagnosis*
- ***Most recent Skin Test: C-Tb (Cytokine-Tuberculosis) Test***
    - *Key Features of the C-Tb Test*
    - *Advantages and Limitations of the C-Tb Test*
    - *Clinical Trials, Current Status & Future of the C-Tb Test*

23. Biomarkers and Serological Tests

- ***Serodiagnostic Tests for TB*** *(Not WHO recommended)*
    - *Antibody-based assays*
    - *Challenges with specificity and sensitivity*
- ***Host Biomarker-Based Tests***
    - *IP-10, TNF-α , and other cytokine-based assays*
    - *Use of transcriptomics and proteomics in TB diagnosis*

24. Radiological and Imaging Techniques in TB Diagnosis

- **Chest X-Ray (CXR) and Scoring Systems**
  - *Features suggestive of active vs. healed TB*
  - *WHO-endorsed AI-assisted CXR interpretation*
- **Computed Tomography (CT) and Magnetic Resonance Imaging (MRI)**
  - *Utility in diagnosing extrapulmonary TB (brain, spine, abdomen)*
- **Ultrasound in TB Diagnosis**
  - *Abdominal TB, lymphadenitis, and pleural effusion assessment*
- **Positron Emission Tomography (PET-CT) in TB**
  - *Emerging role in TB diagnostics and treatment response monitoring*

25. Drug Susceptibility Testing (DST)

- **Phenotypic DST**
  - *Proportion method*
  - *MGIT-based DST*
- **Genotypic DST**
  - *rpoB mutations in rifampicin resistance*
  - *katG and inhA mutations in isoniazid resistance*
  - *gyrA, gyrB mutations in fluoroquinolone resistance*
  - *Second-line DST approaches*

26. Diagnosis of Latent TB Infection (LTBI)

- *Importance in TB control programs*
- *Comparative performance of TST vs. IGRA*
- *Overview & Summary: Which TB Test Should Be Used?*
- *Role of preventive therapy based on diagnostic findings*

27. Diagnosis of Extrapulmonary TB

- ***CNS TB:*** *CSF analysis, ADA, PCR, imaging correlation*
- ***Pleural TB:*** *ADA, LDH, culture, GeneXpert on pleural fluid*
- ***Abdominal TB:*** *FNAC, biopsy, ascitic fluid analysis*
- ***Osteoarticular TB:*** *MRI-guided biopsies, culture, PCR*
- ***Genitourinary TB:*** *Urine TB-PCR, Mycobacterial culture*
- ***Miliary TB:*** *Blood culture, CXR, molecular tests*

Abbreviations

ACF - Active Case Finding
ADA - Adenosine Deaminase
AFB - Acid-Fast Bacilli
AI - Artificial Intelligence
AIDS - Acquired Immunodeficiency Syndrome
ASM - American Society for Microbiology
ATF - Activating Transcription Factor
ATP - Adenosine Triphosphate
BACTEC - Bacteriological Culture System
BCE - Before Common Era
BCG - Bacillus Calmette-Guérin
BR - Biochemical Reactions
BSL - Biosafety Level
CBNAAT - Cartridge-Based Nucleic Acid Amplification Test
CDC - Centers for Disease Control and Prevention
CFP - Culture Filtrate Protein
CNS - Central Nervous System
COVID-19 - Coronavirus Disease 2019
CRISPR - Clustered Regularly Interspaced Short Palindromic Repeats
CT - Computed Tomography
C-Tb - Cytokine-Tuberculosis Test
CXR - Chest X-Ray
DMT - Direct Microscopy Test
DNA - Deoxyribonucleic Acid
DOTS - Directly Observed Treatment, Short-Course
DST - Drug Susceptibility Testing
ECDC - European Centre for Disease Prevention and Control
ELISA - Enzyme-Linked Immunosorbent Assay
EPTB - Extrapulmonary Tuberculosis
ESAT-6 - Early Secretory Antigenic Target-6
FNAC - Fine-Needle Aspiration Cytology
GB - Granulomatous Bacteria
GIT - Gastrointestinal Tract
HIV - Human Immunodeficiency Virus
HRZE - Isoniazid, Rifampicin, Pyrazinamide, Ethambutol (TB Treatment Regimen)
ICMR - Indian Council of Medical Research
IFN-γ - Interferon-Gamma
IGRA - Interferon-Gamma Release Assay
IL-2 - Interleukin-2

IL-6 - Interleukin-6
IP-10 - Interferon-Gamma Inducible Protein 10
LAMP - Loop-Mediated Isothermal Amplification
LAM - Lipoarabinomannan
LJ - Löwenstein-Jensen Medium
LTBI - Latent Tuberculosis Infection
M. tb - Mycobacterium tuberculosis
MGIT - Mycobacteria Growth Indicator Tube
MDR-TB - Multidrug-Resistant Tuberculosis
MRI - Magnetic Resonance Imaging
MTBC - Mycobacterium tuberculosis Complex
NAAT - Nucleic Acid Amplification Test
NGS - Next-Generation Sequencing
NTM - Nontuberculous Mycobacteria
NTEP - National Tuberculosis Elimination Program
PCR - Polymerase Chain Reaction
PET-CT - Positron Emission Tomography-Computed Tomography
PPD - Purified Protein Derivative
QFT - QuantiFERON-TB Test
RNA - Ribonucleic Acid
rpoB - RNA Polymerase Beta Subunit (Gene Associated with Rifampicin Resistance)
SOD - Superoxide Dismutase
TB - Tuberculosis
TBM - Tuberculous Meningitis
TNF-α - Tumor Necrosis Factor-Alpha
TST - Tuberculin Skin Test
WGS - Whole-Genome Sequencing
WHO - World Health Organization
XDR-TB - Extensively Drug-Resistant Tuberculosis

SECTION 1

INTRODUCTION TO MYCOBACTERIUM TUBERCULOSIS

1. Historical Background and Discovery

The discovery of *Mycobacterium tuberculosis* (M. tuberculosis) marked a crucial turning point in medical microbiology. Tuberculosis (TB) has afflicted humanity for thousands of years, with evidence found in Egyptian mummies dating back to 3000 BCE. The disease was historically known by various names, including "consumption" and "phthisis," due to its wasting effects on the body.

The breakthrough came in 1882 when **Dr. Robert Koch**, a German physician and microbiologist, identified *M. tuberculosis* as the causative agent of TB. Using his groundbreaking staining techniques and the principles of germ theory, Koch was able to demonstrate the bacterium under a microscope. His work laid the foundation for modern bacteriology and earned him the **Nobel Prize in Physiology or Medicine** in 1905.

Ancient and Medieval Perspectives on TB

- The disease was known as "Pott's disease" in cases of spinal TB, first described by **Percivall Pott** in the 18th century.
- In ancient Greece, Hippocrates referred to TB as **"phthisis"**, emphasizing its chronic and often fatal nature.
- The Industrial Revolution saw a sharp increase in TB cases due to urban overcrowding, poor hygiene, and malnutrition.

Post-Koch Developments

- Albert Calmette and Camille Guérin developed the **BCG vaccine** in the early 20th century.
- The advent of **streptomycin (1943)** by Selman Waksman and colleagues provided the first effective antibiotic treatment for TB.
- WHO declared TB a global health emergency in 1993 due to rising drug resistance.

2. Evolution and Phylogenetic of M. tuberculosis

M. *tuberculosis* belongs to the **Mycobacterium tuberculosis complex (MTBC)**, a group of closely related species causing TB in humans and animals. Evolutionary studies suggest that M. *tuberculosis* evolved from an environmental mycobacterium millions of years ago and adapted to mammalian hosts.

Key Aspects of M. tuberculosis Evolution

- **Common Ancestor Hypothesis:** Genome sequencing studies indicate that *M. tuberculosis* shares a common ancestor with *Mycobacterium canettii* and other environmental mycobacteria.
- **Clonal Population Structure:** Unlike many bacteria, *M. tuberculosis* has a clonal structure with minimal horizontal gene transfer.
- **Lineage Classification:** *M. tuberculosis* is classified into various lineages based on geographic distribution:
    - **Lineage 1 (Indo-Oceanic)** – Found in Southeast Asia and the Pacific region.
    - **Lineage 2 (East Asian/Beijing strain)** – Highly virulent and associated with drug resistance.
    - **Lineage 3 (East African-Indian)** – Prevalent in India and East Africa.
    - **Lineage 4 (Euro-American)** – The most widespread global lineage.

Genomic Adaptations for Pathogenicity

M. tuberculosis has evolved several genomic features that enhance its ability to infect and persist in hosts:

- **PE/PPE Gene Families:** Encode proteins involved in immune evasion.
- **DosR Regulon:** Enables survival under hypoxic conditions within granulomas.
- **Mutations in Drug Resistance Genes:** Evolutionary adaptations leading to multidrug-resistant (MDR) and extensively drug-resistant (XDR) TB.

3. General Characteristics and Morphology

M. tuberculosis is a unique bacterium with distinct structural and physiological properties that contribute to its pathogenesis.

Morphological Features

- **Shape:** Rod-shaped (bacillus), measuring **2-4 µm in length and 0.2-0.5 µm in width.**
- **Acid-Fastness:** Due to its waxy cell wall, it retains the red stain in Ziehl-Neelsen (ZN) staining despite acid-alcohol treatment.
- **Non-Motile and Non-Spore Forming:** Lacks flagella or pili and does not form spores.
- **Obligate Aerobe:** Requires oxygen for survival and growth.

Growth Characteristics

- **Slow Growth:** Doubling time of **15-20 hours**, much slower than many bacterial pathogens.
- **Colony Morphology:** Forms rough, buff-colored colonies on Löwenstein-Jensen (LJ) medium.
- **Temperature Requirements:** Grows optimally at **37°C**, consistent with human body temperature.

Staining and Identification

M. *tuberculosis* is identified using:

- **Ziehl-Neelsen Staining:** Detects acid-fast bacilli (AFB) in clinical samples.
- **Fluorescent Microscopy (Auramine-Rhodamine Staining):** More sensitive than ZN staining.
- **Gram Stain:** Poorly stains due to high lipid content in the cell wall.

4. Cell Wall Composition and Its Role in Pathogenicity

The **unique cell wall structure** of M. *tuberculosis* is crucial for its survival, virulence, and resistance to host immune responses and antibiotics.

Key Components of the M. tuberculosis Cell Wall

1. **Peptidoglycan Layer**
   - Provides structural integrity and maintains cell shape.
2. **Arabinogalactan Layer**
   - Bridges peptidoglycan and mycolic acids.
3. **Mycolic Acids**
   - Long-chain fatty acids that form a hydrophobic barrier, making the cell wall highly impermeable.
4. **Lipoarabinomannan (LAM)**
   - Inhibits immune responses by blocking T-cell activation and inducing macrophage apoptosis.
5. **Phthiocerol Dimycocerosates (PDIMs)**
   - Contribute to virulence by preventing phagosome-lysosome fusion.
6. **Trehalose Dimycolate (TDM or Cord Factor)**
   - Key virulence factor causing granuloma formation and immune modulation.

Role in Pathogenesis

- **Resistance to Antibiotics:** The lipid-rich cell wall reduces permeability to hydrophilic drugs, contributing to natural drug resistance.
- **Immune Evasion:** LAM and PDIMs allow the bacterium to survive within macrophages.
- **Persistence in Host:** Slow-growing nature and dormancy-inducing mechanisms enable latent TB infection (LTBI).

Conclusion

The understanding of *Mycobacterium tuberculosis* at a historical, evolutionary, morphological, and structural level is fundamental to developing effective diagnostic, therapeutic, and preventive strategies. The unique characteristics of *M. tuberculosis*, particularly its slow growth, complex cell wall, and immune evasion mechanisms, make TB a challenging disease to control. Future research into its evolutionary adaptations and resistance mechanisms will be critical for global TB eradication efforts.

SECTION 2

EPIDEMIOLOGY AND PUBLIC HEALTH

5. Global and Regional Burden of Tuberculosis (TB)

Tuberculosis remains one of the deadliest infectious diseases worldwide. According to the World Health Organization (WHO), TB caused an estimated 10 million new infections and 1.5 million deaths in 2020. The disease disproportionately affects low- and middle-income countries, particularly in Asia and Africa.

Global TB Burden

- **High-Burden Countries:** India, China, Indonesia, the Philippines, Pakistan, Nigeria, Bangladesh, and South Africa account for the majority of TB cases.
- **Drug-Resistant TB:** Multidrug-resistant TB (MDR-TB) and extensively drug-resistant TB (XDR-TB) pose significant public health challenges.
- **TB and HIV Co-Infection:** TB is the leading cause of death among people living with HIV/AIDS.
- **WHO End TB Strategy:** Aims to reduce TB deaths by 90% and new cases by 80% by 2030.

Regional TB Epidemiology

- **South Asia:** India bears the highest TB burden globally, with an estimated 2.6 million cases annually.
- **Africa:** High prevalence due to HIV co-infection, malnutrition, and poor healthcare infrastructure.
- **Europe and North America:** Lower TB incidence, but rising cases of drug-resistant TB.
- **Latin America:** Intermediate burden with high urban transmission rates.

6. Transmission Dynamics and Risk Factors

TB is primarily transmitted via airborne droplets expelled when an infected person coughs, sneezes, or talks. The probability of transmission depends on various factors:

Modes of Transmission

- **Droplet Nuclei:** Small particles (1–5 microns) containing *M. tuberculosis* remain airborne for hours.
- **Close Contact Exposure:** Family members, healthcare workers, and coworkers are at higher risk.
- **Fomites and Surface Contamination:** Not a major route but possible in clinical settings.

Key Risk Factors

- **Immunocompromised States:** HIV infection, diabetes mellitus, malnutrition, and immunosuppressive therapy increase susceptibility.
- **Socioeconomic Factors:** Poverty, overcrowding, and poor ventilation facilitate transmission.
- **Occupational Exposure:** Healthcare workers, miners, and prison populations face higher risks.
- **Substance Abuse:** Smoking and alcohol use disorder contribute to increased TB risk.
- **Genetic Susceptibility:** Certain genetic polymorphisms affect TB susceptibility and progression.

7. Latent vs. Active TB Infection

TB exists in two forms: **latent TB infection (LTBI)** and **active TB disease.**

Latent TB Infection (LTBI)

- Individuals are infected with *M. tuberculosis* but show no symptoms.
- The immune system contains the infection, preventing progression.
- Diagnosis: Tuberculin Skin Test (TST) and Interferon-Gamma Release Assays (IGRAs).
- Treatment: Isoniazid (INH) preventive therapy (IPT) or rifapentine-based regimens.

Active TB Disease

- Occurs when *M. tuberculosis* overcomes immune control.
- Symptoms: Persistent cough, fever, night sweats, weight loss, hemoptysis.
- Diagnosis: Sputum smear microscopy, molecular tests (GeneXpert), and culture.
- Treatment: Standard 6-month regimen (HRZE: Isoniazid, Rifampicin, Pyrazinamide, Ethambutol).

Progression from Latent to Active TB

- Approximately **5-10%** of LTBI cases progress to active TB.
- **Higher Risk Groups:** HIV-positive individuals, diabetics, transplant patients, and individuals on prolonged corticosteroid therapy.

8. Socioeconomic and Environmental Influences on TB Spread

The burden of TB is closely linked to **social determinants of health.** Addressing these factors is essential for TB control.

Impact of Poverty on TB

- **Malnutrition:** Weakens the immune system, increasing TB susceptibility.
- **Overcrowded Housing:** Facilitates airborne transmission, especially in urban slums and refugee camps.
- **Limited Access to Healthcare:** Delays diagnosis and treatment, leading to increased spread.
- **Financial Burden of TB Treatment:** Despite free treatment in many countries, indirect costs (transport, loss of income) remain significant.

Environmental Factors in TB Transmission

- **Air Pollution:** Inhalation of pollutants weakens lung defences.
- **Indoor Air Quality:** Poor ventilation increases transmission risks.
- **Climate Change:** Changing weather patterns may influence TB epidemiology.

TB and Migration

- **Refugees and Migrant Populations:** Often have limited access to healthcare, increasing the risk of undiagnosed and untreated TB.
- **TB Screening at Borders:** Some countries implement TB testing for immigrants to prevent the spread of drug-resistant strains.

Community-Based TB Control Measures

- **Active Case Finding (ACF):** Identifying TB cases through community outreach.
- **DOTS Strategy:** Directly observed therapy short-course to ensure treatment adherence.
- **Public Awareness Campaigns:** Educating communities about TB transmission and prevention.

Conclusion

Epidemiology plays a crucial role in understanding and controlling TB. The global burden of TB remains high, particularly in developing countries, where social determinants contribute to its spread. Effective TB control requires a **multi-sectoral approach** integrating healthcare, socio-economic interventions, and public health policies. Strengthening diagnostic capabilities, improving access to treatment, and addressing risk factors will be key to achieving the **End TB Strategy goals by 2030.**

SECTION 3

PATHOGENESIS AND IMMUNOLOGY

9. Host-Pathogen Interaction

Tuberculosis (TB) is caused by *Mycobacterium tuberculosis* (M. tuberculosis), an intracellular pathogen that primarily infects alveolar macrophages in the lungs. The host-pathogen interaction in TB is a complex process involving immune evasion strategies, granuloma formation, and host immune responses that determine disease progression.

Stages of Infection

1. **Entry and Initial Infection**
    - Inhalation of *M. tuberculosis* bacilli in airborne droplets.
    - Bacilli reach the alveoli and are phagocytosed by alveolar macrophages.
2. **Intracellular Survival and Immune Evasion**
    - *M. tuberculosis* inhibits phagosome-lysosome fusion, preventing bacterial degradation.
    - Secretion of proteins (e.g., ESAT-6, CFP-10) disrupts host immune signaling.
3. **Granuloma Formation**
    - Macrophages recruit T cells, dendritic cells, and neutrophils to form granulomas.
    - Granulomas contain the infection but also serve as reservoirs for latent TB.
4. **Reactivation and Dissemination**
    - If the immune system weakens, granulomas break down, leading to active TB.
    - *M. tuberculosis* spreads to other organs via the bloodstream.

10. Mechanisms of Immune Evasion by M. tuberculosis

M. tuberculosis has evolved multiple strategies to evade host immunity and persist within macrophages.

Key Immune Evasion Strategies

1. **Inhibition of Phagosome Maturation**
    - *M. tuberculosis* secretes PknG, SapM, and TACO to block phagosome-lysosome fusion.
    - Bacilli remain within an immature phagosome, avoiding degradation.
2. **Suppression of Antigen Presentation**
    - Downregulation of MHC-II molecules reduces T-cell activation.

- Inhibition of dendritic cell maturation limits adaptive immune responses.

3. **Modulation of Host Cell Death Pathways**
   - Inhibition of apoptosis allows bacterial survival within host cells.
   - Induction of necrosis promotes bacterial release and further infection.
4. **Resistance to Reactive Oxygen and Nitrogen Species (ROS/RNS)**
   - Expression of KatG (catalase-peroxidase) detoxifies reactive oxygen species.
   - Superoxide dismutase (SOD) neutralizes oxidative stress within macrophages.

11. Granuloma Formation and Disease Progression

Granulomas are organized immune structures that serve as the hallmark of TB infection.

Formation and Function of Granulomas

1. **Early Granuloma Formation**
   - Macrophages engulf *M. tuberculosis* and secrete chemokines (CCL2, CXCL10) to recruit immune cells.
   - Infected macrophages differentiate into foamy macrophages and multinucleated giant cells.
2. **Mature Granuloma Structure**
   - Core: Infected macrophages, foamy macrophages, and necrotic debris.
   - Middle layer: T cells (CD4+, CD8+), dendritic cells, and fibroblasts.
   - Outer layer: Fibrotic tissue and regulatory immune cells.
3. **Necrosis and Cavitation**
   - Caseous necrosis forms due to immune-mediated tissue damage.
   - If granulomas rupture, *M. tuberculosis* spreads, leading to active TB.

12. Role of Cytokines and Immune Cells in TB

Cytokines play a crucial role in the immune response to *M. tuberculosis*.

Key Cytokines in TB Immunity

1. **Interferon-Gamma (IFN-γ)**
   - Produced by Th1 cells to activate macrophages.
   - Enhances production of reactive nitrogen species (RNS) to kill bacteria.

2. **Tumor Necrosis Factor-Alpha (TNF-α)**
    - Promotes granuloma maintenance and macrophage activation.
    - Excess TNF-α causes tissue damage and contributes to caseation necrosis.
3. **Interleukin-10 (IL-10)**
    - Inhibits pro-inflammatory responses, leading to bacterial persistence.
    - Suppresses antigen presentation and reduces IFN-γ production.
4. **Interleukin-12 (IL-12)**
    - Enhances Th1 differentiation and IFN-γ production.
    - Essential for resistance against *M. tuberculosis* infection.

Role of Immune Cells

1. **Macrophages**
    - First line of defense; phagocytose *M. tuberculosis* but may become reservoirs for bacterial persistence.
2. **Dendritic Cells**
    - Present antigens to naive T cells, initiating adaptive immune responses.
3. **T Cells**
    - **CD4+ T Cells (Th1 subtype):** Produce IFN-γ and activate macrophages.
    - **CD8+ T Cells:** Kill infected macrophages and secrete perforins.
4. **Neutrophils**
    - Contribute to early infection control but also cause tissue damage.
5. **Regulatory T Cells (Tregs)**
    - Suppress immune activation and contribute to chronic infection.

Conclusion

Understanding the pathogenesis and immunology of *M. tuberculosis* is critical for developing novel therapeutics and vaccines. The interaction between the pathogen and the host immune system determines the outcome of infection, from latent TB to active disease. Ongoing research on immune evasion mechanisms, granuloma biology, and cytokine networks will enhance TB control strategies and improve treatment outcomes.

SECTION 4

CLINICAL MANIFESTATIONS OF TUBERCULOSIS

Introduction

Tuberculosis (TB) presents in multiple clinical forms, each with its own unique challenges in diagnosis and management. Understanding these manifestations is crucial for timely detection and effective treatment. This section comprehensively explores the clinical presentation of pulmonary TB, extrapulmonary TB, pediatric TB, and TB-HIV co-infection.

13. Pulmonary Tuberculosis – Symptoms and Diagnosis

Pulmonary tuberculosis (PTB) is the most common and contagious form of the disease, primarily affecting the lungs. Its clinical spectrum ranges from mild to severe symptoms, depending on the host's immune response and bacterial load.

Symptoms of Pulmonary TB

1. **Persistent Cough:** Lasting more than three weeks, initially dry but eventually productive with sputum, sometimes blood-tinged (hemoptysis).
2. **Fever and Night Sweats:** A low-grade fever that typically worsens in the evening and is associated with night sweats.
3. **Weight Loss and Anorexia:** Progressive loss of appetite and unintended weight loss due to systemic effects of TB.
4. **Chest Pain:** Often pleuritic in nature, worsening with deep breathing.
5. **Fatigue and Malaise:** Generalized weakness due to chronic infection.
6. **Dyspnea (Shortness of Breath):** In advanced cases due to extensive lung damage.

Diagnosis of Pulmonary TB

1. **Sputum Microscopy (Acid-Fast Bacillus Staining):** A simple and widely used test, though it lacks sensitivity in paucibacillary cases.
2. **Culture Techniques:** Gold standard for TB diagnosis, with MGIT (Mycobacteria Growth Indicator Tube) and Löwenstein-Jensen medium being commonly used.
3. **Molecular Diagnostics:** GeneXpert MTB/RIF and Line Probe Assay (LPA) for rapid detection and drug resistance profiling.
4. **Radiographic Imaging:** Chest X-ray and CT scans revealing cavitations, nodules, or miliary TB patterns.
5. **Tuberculin Skin Test (TST) and IGRA:** Supporting tools for identifying latent TB infections.

14. Extrapulmonary TB – Types and Clinical Features

Extrapulmonary tuberculosis (EPTB) occurs when Mycobacterium tuberculosis spreads beyond the lungs, affecting other organs.

Common Forms of Extrapulmonary TB

1. **Lymph Node TB (Tuberculous Lymphadenitis):**
    - Most common form of EPTB.
    - Presents with painless swelling of lymph nodes, usually in the cervical region.
    - Diagnosis via fine-needle aspiration cytology (FNAC) or excisional biopsy.
2. **Pleural TB:**
    - Symptoms include pleuritic chest pain, breathlessness, and pleural effusion.
    - Diagnosed by pleural fluid analysis and adenosine deaminase (ADA) testing.
3. **Abdominal TB:**
    - Involves the intestines, peritoneum, or solid organs.
    - Symptoms include abdominal pain, weight loss, diarrhea, and ascites.
    - Diagnosed using ultrasound-guided biopsy and laparoscopic examination.
4. **Skeletal TB:**
    - Affects the spine (Pott's disease) and joints.
    - Manifests as chronic back pain, deformity, and neurological deficits.
    - MRI is the preferred diagnostic tool.
5. **Central Nervous System (CNS) TB:**
    - Includes tuberculous meningitis, brain abscesses, and spinal cord involvement.
    - Symptoms: headache, neck stiffness, altered mental status, seizures.
    - Diagnosed via cerebrospinal fluid (CSF) analysis, imaging, and PCR-based tests.
6. **Genitourinary TB:**
    - Affects the kidneys, bladder, and reproductive organs.
    - Presents with hematuria, flank pain, infertility in women.
    - Diagnosed by urine culture and PCR.

15. Pediatric Tuberculosis

TB in children presents differently from adults, often posing a diagnostic challenge due to non-specific symptoms.

Common Clinical Features in Pediatric TB

1. **Primary TB Complex:**
   - Includes mild fever, cough, and lymphadenopathy.
   - Often asymptomatic, detected through contact screening.
2. **Progressive Primary TB:**
   - Severe cases with bronchopneumonia-like symptoms, weight loss, and failure to thrive.
3. **Miliary TB:**
   - Disseminated form with widespread TB lesions.
   - Presents with respiratory distress, hepatosplenomegaly, and high fever.
4. **Tuberculous Meningitis:**
   - Serious form leading to neurological complications.
   - Symptoms include irritability, vomiting, convulsions, and altered sensorium.

Diagnosis in Children

1. **Gastric Aspirate & Induced Sputum:** Since young children rarely produce sputum.
2. **TST & IGRA:** More reliable than sputum microscopy.
3. **Chest X-ray:** Identifies primary complex or miliary TB patterns.
4. **Molecular Tests (Xpert MTB/RIF):** Increasingly used for rapid diagnosis.

16. TB and HIV Co-Infection

TB is a leading cause of morbidity and mortality in people living with HIV (PLHIV). The interaction between TB and HIV accelerates disease progression.

Clinical Features of TB-HIV Co-Infection

1. **Atypical TB Presentation:**
   - More extrapulmonary and disseminated forms.
   - Less cavitary lung disease; more interstitial and military patterns.
2. **Severe Immunosuppression Symptoms:**

    - Wasting syndrome, persistent diarrhea, and generalized lymphadenopathy.
3. **Paradoxical TB-IRIS (Immune Reconstitution Inflammatory Syndrome):**
    - Exacerbation of TB symptoms after starting antiretroviral therapy (ART).

Diagnosis in HIV-TB Co-Infection

1. **Sputum Smear & Culture:** Often negative due to lower bacillary load.
2. **GeneXpert MTB/RIF:** Recommended due to higher sensitivity in HIV-positive individuals.
3. **Urine Lipoarabinomannan (LAM) Test:** Rapid diagnostic tool useful in severely immunocompromised patients.
4. **Chest X-ray & CT Scans:** Helps in detecting atypical TB patterns.

Management and Treatment Considerations

- **Concurrent TB and HIV Treatment:** ART should be initiated in all HIV-positive TB patients, but timing varies depending on severity.
- **Drug-Drug Interactions:** Rifampicin interacts with antiretroviral drugs, requiring dose adjustments.
- **Preventive Therapy:** Isoniazid preventive therapy (IPT) recommended for high-risk groups.

Conclusion

Understanding the diverse clinical presentations of TB is essential for accurate diagnosis and effective treatment. Pulmonary and extrapulmonary TB manifest differently, requiring tailored diagnostic strategies. Pediatric TB poses unique challenges, necessitating specialized approaches. TB-HIV co-infection remains a major public health concern, demanding integrated care strategies. Addressing these complexities is key to improving global TB control and patient outcomes.

SECTION 5

LABORATORY DIAGNOSIS OF TUBERCULOSIS

17. General Principles of TB Diagnosis

Importance of Early and Accurate Diagnosis

Tuberculosis (TB) is one of the top infectious disease killers worldwide, responsible for significant morbidity and mortality. Early and accurate diagnosis of TB is critical for reducing transmission, initiating appropriate treatment, and preventing complications such as drug resistance. Diagnosis plays a crucial role in global TB control strategies, as untreated TB patients serve as reservoirs for continued disease transmission.

Benefits of Early Detection

- **Reduces transmission:** TB spreads through airborne droplets, and early diagnosis helps isolate infectious patients to prevent further spread.
- **Improves treatment outcomes:** Delayed diagnosis is associated with increased lung damage, prolonged illness, and higher mortality rates.
- **Prevents complications:** TB can disseminate beyond the lungs, leading to extrapulmonary TB, which can be life-threatening if not diagnosed in time.
- **Reduces the burden on healthcare systems:** Prompt diagnosis and treatment lower hospitalization rates and healthcare costs.
- **Facilitates public health interventions:** Early case detection allows contact tracing and preventive treatment for at-risk populations.

Role of Laboratory Diagnosis in TB Control

While clinical symptoms like chronic cough, weight loss, and fever raise suspicion of TB, laboratory tests provide definitive confirmation. Laboratory methods range from traditional techniques like microscopy and culture to advanced molecular diagnostics, which enable rapid and accurate detection.

Challenges in TB Diagnosis

Despite advancements in TB diagnostics, several challenges persist, impacting timely and accurate detection of the disease.

Low Bacterial Load and Smear-Negative TB

- Sputum smear microscopy remains a primary diagnostic tool in many settings, but its sensitivity is limited.
- Patients with early-stage TB or extrapulmonary TB often have low bacterial loads, making microscopy-based diagnosis challenging.

- HIV-associated TB cases frequently present with smear-negative disease, necessitating more sensitive diagnostic tools like culture or nucleic acid amplification tests (NAATs).

Extrapulmonary TB (EPTB) Diagnosis

- TB can affect organs outside the lungs, including the lymph nodes, pleura, bones, joints, meninges, and the genitourinary system.
- Extrapulmonary samples (e.g., cerebrospinal fluid, pleural fluid, biopsy specimens) typically have lower bacillary loads, making detection more difficult.
- Invasive procedures, such as biopsies or fine-needle aspiration, are required to obtain suitable samples, adding complexity to the diagnostic process.

Drug-Resistant TB (DR-TB) Detection

- Multidrug-resistant TB (MDR-TB) and extensively drug-resistant TB (XDR-TB) pose serious threats to TB control.
- Conventional culture-based drug susceptibility testing (DST) takes weeks, delaying appropriate treatment initiation.
- Rapid molecular tests like GeneXpert MTB/RIF and line-probe assays have improved early DR-TB detection but are not universally available.
- Access to second-line DST for drugs like fluoroquinolones and bedaquiline remains limited in many high-burden countries.

Diagnostic Gaps in Low-Resource Settings

- Many high TB-burden countries face challenges in accessing advanced diagnostic tools due to financial constraints and weak laboratory infrastructure.
- Availability of rapid molecular tests is limited in rural areas, where most TB cases are diagnosed using conventional microscopy.
- Long turnaround times for culture-based diagnostics hinder timely initiation of treatment.
- Lack of trained personnel for performing and interpreting complex diagnostic tests.

WHO Guidelines and Diagnostic Algorithms

The World Health Organization (WHO) provides global guidance on TB diagnosis, emphasizing the need for rapid, accurate, and accessible tests to improve case detection and treatment outcomes.

WHO Recommended Diagnostic Approaches

The WHO recommends a multi-pronged approach for TB diagnosis, incorporating microbiological, molecular, and immunological tests:

- **Microscopy-based methods:** Ziehl-Neelsen (ZN) staining and LED fluorescence microscopy (FM) for acid-fast bacilli (AFB) detection.
- **Culture-based methods:** Solid (Löwenstein-Jensen) and liquid (MGIT 960) culture systems for mycobacterial growth and DST.
- **Molecular tests:** GeneXpert MTB/RIF and Truenat for rapid TB and rifampicin resistance detection.
- **Immunodiagnostic tests:** Interferon-gamma release assays (IGRAs) and tuberculin skin test (TST) for latent TB infection (LTBI) screening.
- **Whole-genome sequencing (WGS):** Used for drug resistance profiling and epidemiological surveillance in advanced settings.

WHO Diagnostic Algorithm for Pulmonary TB

The WHO recommends the following steps for diagnosing pulmonary TB:

1. **Initial assessment:** Symptom screening (cough >2 weeks, fever, weight loss, night sweats, hemoptysis).
2. **Microscopy or molecular testing:** GeneXpert MTB/RIF as the preferred initial test in all patients with presumptive TB.
3. **Culture and DST:** If GeneXpert MTB/RIF is unavailable or inconclusive, perform sputum culture and DST.
4. **Chest X-ray (CXR):** Used as a supplementary tool to detect lung abnormalities.
5. **Further evaluation for DR-TB:** If rifampicin resistance is detected, second-line DST should be conducted.

WHO Algorithm for Extrapulmonary TB Diagnosis

Diagnosis of EPTB depends on the affected organ system and requires a combination of clinical, radiological, and laboratory investigations:

1. **Clinical suspicion:** Based on symptoms such as lymphadenopathy, meningitis, pleural effusion, joint pain, or genitourinary symptoms.
2. **Sample collection:** Fine-needle aspiration, pleural fluid tapping, CSF collection, or biopsy.
3. **Microbiological testing:** GeneXpert MTB/RIF is recommended for CSF, lymph node, and pleural fluid samples.
4. **Histopathology:** Biopsy specimens may show granulomatous inflammation with caseous necrosis.
5. **Adjunct imaging:** MRI, CT, or ultrasound can aid in localizing TB lesions.

WHO Recommendations for Drug-Resistant TB Detection

1. **Universal DST:** WHO recommends DST for all diagnosed TB cases to detect drug resistance early.
2. **First-line DST:** GeneXpert MTB/RIF or line-probe assays should be performed to detect rifampicin and isoniazid resistance.
3. **Second-line DST:** For MDR-TB cases, further testing for fluoroquinolones and second-line injectable drugs is necessary.
4. **Whole-genome sequencing (WGS):** Used for detailed drug resistance profiling and outbreak investigations.

Role of Artificial Intelligence (AI) in TB Diagnosis

- AI-assisted interpretation of chest X-rays (e.g., CAD4TB) enhances TB screening in high-burden areas.
- Digital microscopy with AI algorithms improves the accuracy of smear microscopy.
- AI-driven diagnostic platforms integrate multiple test results to improve clinical decision-making.

18. Sample Collection and Processing

Accurate diagnosis of tuberculosis (TB) relies heavily on proper sample collection and processing. The quality and integrity of the specimens play a crucial role in determining the sensitivity and specificity of diagnostic tests. This section outlines the principles, methods, and best practices for collecting and processing samples for pulmonary, extrapulmonary, and latent TB diagnosis, along with considerations for biosafety and transportation.

Pulmonary TB: Sputum Collection Techniques

Pulmonary TB is the most common form of tuberculosis, and sputum remains the primary diagnostic specimen. Proper collection techniques significantly impact test accuracy, particularly for smear microscopy, culture, and molecular diagnostics.

Sputum Collection Techniques

A. Spot and Morning Sputum Collection

The World Health Organization (WHO) recommends two specimens—one early morning and one spot sputum sample—to optimize the detection rate of Mycobacterium tuberculosis.

- **Morning Sputum Collection:**
    - Collected immediately upon waking up, before eating or drinking.
    - Higher bacterial load due to overnight accumulation in the lungs.
    - Increases sensitivity of smear microscopy and molecular tests.
- **Spot Sputum Collection:**
    - Obtained at the healthcare facility during the patient's visit.
    - Ensures a sample is collected even if the patient does not return for a morning specimen.
    - Typically used for GeneXpert MTB/RIF testing, where one good-quality sample is often sufficient.

B. Induced Sputum Collection

Some TB suspects, particularly children and patients with HIV or other immunocompromised conditions, may be unable to produce sputum spontaneously. Induced sputum collection involves inhalation of a saline or hypertonic saline mist to stimulate sputum production.

- **Procedure:**
    1. The patient inhales nebulized sterile hypertonic saline (3–5%) for 15–20 minutes.
    2. Sputum is expectorated into a sterile container under supervision.
    3. If expectoration is inadequate, gentle chest physiotherapy may assist in sputum production.
- **Advantages:**
    - Non-invasive alternative to bronchoscopy.
    - Higher diagnostic yield compared to expectorated sputum.
- **Challenges:**
    - Requires trained personnel and nebulization equipment.
    - Increased risk of nosocomial transmission if biosafety precautions are not followed.

Extrapulmonary TB: Sample Types

Extrapulmonary TB (EPTB) accounts for a significant proportion of TB cases, especially in immunocompromised individuals. The choice of specimen depends on the site of infection. The following are key sample types and collection methods for EPTB diagnosis:

Cerebrospinal Fluid (CSF) Collection for TB Meningitis

- **Indication:** TB meningitis (TBM), a severe form of EPTB, requires CSF examination.
- **Procedure:**
    1. Collected via lumbar puncture under sterile conditions.
    2. At least 5–10 mL of CSF is required for testing.
    3. Should be processed immediately for microscopy, culture, and GeneXpert MTB/RIF.
- **Findings:** Elevated protein, low glucose, and lymphocytic pleocytosis in CSF analysis support TBM diagnosis.

Pleural Fluid for TB Pleuritis

- **Indication:** TB pleuritis, characterized by pleural effusion.
- **Procedure:**
    1. Collected via thoracentesis using aseptic technique.
    2. Minimum 50 mL required for culture and biochemical analysis.
- **Findings:**
    - High adenosine deaminase (ADA) (>40 IU/L) suggests TB.

- Culture yield is low; GeneXpert or histopathology of pleural biopsy may be more effective.

Fine-Needle Aspiration Cytology (FNAC) for Lymph Node TB

- **Indication:** TB lymphadenitis (scrofula) affects cervical, axillary, or inguinal nodes.
- **Procedure:**
  1. Fine-needle aspiration (FNA) is performed using a 22–25-gauge needle.
  2. Sample prepared for smear microscopy, culture, and GeneXpert testing.
- **Findings:** Granulomatous inflammation with caseation necrosis is highly suggestive of TB.

Tissue Biopsy for TB Diagnosis

- **Indication:** TB of bone, intestine, or genitourinary tract.
- **Procedure:**
  1. Collected during surgery or endoscopic procedures.
  2. Tissue samples should be sent for histopathology and microbiological testing.
- **Findings:** Caseating granulomas on histopathology support the diagnosis.

Urine and Blood Samples

- **Indication:** Miliary TB, renal TB.
- **Findings:** Culture positivity in blood or urine suggests disseminated TB.

Latent TB: Blood and Skin-Based Tests

Tuberculin Skin Test (TST)

- **Procedure:**
  1. Intradermal injection of 0.1 mL of purified protein derivative (PPD) on the forearm.
  2. Induration measured after 48–72 hours.
- **Interpretation:**
  - ≥10 mm induration: Positive in most individuals.
  - ≥5 mm in HIV-positive or immunocompromised patients.
- **Limitations:** False positives due to BCG vaccination or non-tuberculous mycobacteria (NTM) exposure.

Interferon-Gamma Release Assays (IGRAs)

- **Types:** QuantiFERON-TB Gold (QFT-GIT), T-SPOT.TB.
- **Advantages:**
    - No cross-reactivity with BCG.
    - Single visit, eliminating need for follow-up.

Sample Transportation and Biosafety Consideration

Proper sample handling and biosafety are critical to prevent contamination and laboratory-acquired infections.

Biosafety Measures

- **Personal Protective Equipment (PPE):** N95 masks, gloves, and lab coats.
- **Biosafety Level 2 (BSL-2) or BSL-3 containment:** Required for handling cultures and aerosol-generating procedures.

Sample Transportation

- **Triple Packaging System:**
    1. Primary container: Leak-proof, labeled specimen container.
    2. Secondary container: Sealed, durable transport tube.
    3. Outer container: Rigid box with absorbent material.
- **Temperature Considerations:**
    - Refrigeration (4°C) for culture samples.
    - Room temperature for smear microscopy.
    - Frozen (-20°C) for molecular testing if delayed.

19. Microscopy-Based Diagnostics

Microscopy remains one of the most widely used diagnostic methods for tuberculosis due to its affordability and rapid turnaround time. Despite its limitations in sensitivity, it plays a crucial role in resource-limited settings. This section covers various microscopy-based methods, including Ziehl-Neelsen (ZN) staining, fluorescent microscopy using auramine-rhodamine staining, and LED fluorescent microscopy.

A. Ziehl-Neelsen (ZN) Staining

Principle

Ziehl-Neelsen (ZN) staining is based on the acid-fast property of Mycobacterium tuberculosis (MTB). The bacterial cell wall contains mycolic acids, which resist decolorization by acid-alcohol after staining with carbol fuchsin, making them appear bright red against a blue background when viewed under a light microscope.

Procedure

1. **Smear Preparation:** A sputum or clinical specimen is spread thinly on a glass slide, air-dried, and heat-fixed.
2. **Staining:**
    - Flood slide with carbol fuchsin and heat gently until steaming for 5 minutes.
    - Rinse with water and decolorize with acid-alcohol for 3 minutes.
    - Counterstain with methylene blue for 30 seconds.
3. **Microscopy Examination:**
    - Observe under an oil immersion objective (1000x magnification).
    - Acid-fast bacilli (AFB) appear red against a blue background.

Interpretation

- **Positive:** Red, beaded, rod-shaped bacilli.
- **Negative:** Absence of AFB in 100 high-power fields.
- **Scanty positive:** 1-9 bacilli per 100 fields.

Limitations

- Requires high bacterial load (~10,000 AFB/mL) for detection.
- Low sensitivity (~50-60%), especially in paucibacillary cases.

- Cannot differentiate MTB from non-tuberculous mycobacteria (NTM).

B. Fluorescent Microscopy (Auramine-Rhodamine Staining)

Sensitivity Comparison with ZN Staining

Fluorescent microscopy using auramine-rhodamine staining is more sensitive (~10% higher) than ZN staining, as fluorescent dyes bind to mycolic acids, making bacilli more visible under a fluorescent microscope.

Procedure

1. **Smear Preparation:** Same as for ZN staining.
2. **Staining:**
    - Flood slide with auramine-rhodamine stain for 10 minutes.
    - Rinse with water and decolorize with acid-alcohol.
    - Counterstain with potassium permanganate for 1 minute.
3. **Microscopy Examination:**
    - Observe under a fluorescent microscope at 400x magnification.
    - AFB appear bright yellow-orange against a dark background.

Advantages in High-Burden Settings

- Faster screening due to low magnification requirement.
- Increased sensitivity (~70-80%).
- Suitable for large-scale TB control programs.

Limitations

- Requires a fluorescent microscope, which is costlier than light microscopes.
- Photobleaching of dyes can affect long-term slide storage.

C. LED Fluorescent Microscopy

WHO Recommendations and Field Applications

The WHO recommends LED-based fluorescent microscopy as a replacement for conventional ZN and auramine-rhodamine methods in high-burden settings. LED microscopy offers advantages such as:

- Comparable sensitivity to auramine-rhodamine staining.
- Longer bulb lifespan (~50,000 hours compared to conventional mercury lamps).

- Low maintenance and energy-efficient.
- Suitable for peripheral laboratories with limited resources.

Detailed Analysis of LED Microscopy

1. Comparison with Conventional Fluorescent Microscopy:

- Unlike mercury vapor lamps, LED microscopy does not require frequent lamp replacements.
- LED sources provide stable illumination, reducing variability in results.

2. Implementation in Resource-Limited Settings:

- LED microscopes can be operated on battery power, making them ideal for remote areas.
- Minimal infrastructure is needed, allowing easy integration into TB diagnostic centers.

3. Studies Supporting LED Microscopy:

- Several field studies have demonstrated that LED microscopy increases TB detection rates by 10-15% over ZN staining.
- WHO-endorsed trials confirm that LED microscopy improves diagnostic accuracy without significant additional costs.

Conclusion

Microscopy-based diagnostics remain crucial in TB detection, particularly in resource-constrained areas. While ZN staining is widely used, fluorescent microscopy and LED fluorescence offer improved sensitivity and faster processing times. Integrating these methods into routine diagnostics can enhance early TB detection and treatment initiation.

D. FLUORESCEIN DIACETATE (FDA) STAINING IN TUBERCULOSIS DIAGNOSIS

Distinguishing between viable and dead *Mycobacterium tuberculosis* (M. tuberculosis) bacilli in sputum smears remains a significant challenge in TB diagnosis and treatment monitoring. Traditional diagnostic methods such as Ziehl-Neelsen (ZN) staining, Auramine-Rhodamine (AR) fluorescent microscopy, and molecular tests like CBNAAT and Line Probe Assay (LPA) detect the presence of TB bacilli but do not differentiate between viable and non-viable organisms.

Fluorescein Diacetate (FDA) staining, a viability-based technique first described over 30 years ago for *M. leprae*, non-tuberculous mycobacteria (MOTT), and *M. tuberculosis*, offers a rapid and cost-effective method to assess bacillary viability in peripheral laboratories. The FDA staining method has gained renewed interest for its potential role in assessing treatment response, guiding drug resistance management, and minimizing unnecessary retreatments.

Principle of FDA Staining

FDA is a fluorogenic substrate that penetrates bacterial cells and is hydrolyzed by intracellular esterases into fluorescein, producing green fluorescence in viable bacilli under fluorescence microscopy. Dead bacilli lack enzymatic activity and fail to fluoresce, appearing FDA-negative.

Advantages of FDA Staining Over Conventional Tests

- **Differentiation Between Live and Dead Bacilli:** Unlike ZN and AR staining, which detect all bacilli irrespective of viability, FDA staining selectively highlights viable *M. tuberculosis*.
- **Rapid Identification of Treatment Response:** FDA-negative smears in ZN-positive patients indicate the presence of non-viable bacilli, helping to determine treatment efficacy.
- **Potential Role in Drug-Resistant TB (DR-TB) Follow-Up:** FDA staining can replace or complement MGIT liquid culture for early identification of treatment failure and resistance.
- **Cost-Effective:** FDA staining is comparable in price to Fluorescent or ZN staining and does not require extensive laboratory infrastructure.
- **Ease of Implementation in Peripheral Laboratories:** Designated Microscopy Centres (DMCs) equipped with LED fluorescent microscopes can integrate FDA staining with minimal training for laboratory technicians.

Clinical Applications of FDA Staining

Treatment Monitoring in TB Patients

- Patients undergoing **anti-tuberculosis treatment (ATT)** are traditionally monitored using sputum smear microscopy and culture.
- FDA staining can help distinguish patients with persistent bacilli that are **viable** from those with **dead bacilli**, reducing the risk of overtreatment and unnecessary changes in regimen.

- At the end of the **Intensive Phase (IP)** and **Continuation Phase (CP)**, FDA-negative results in ZN-positive patients suggest successful treatment response.

Role in Retreatment TB Cases

- Retreatment cases include relapses, treatment after failure, or loss to follow-up on first-line regimens.
- Since CBNAAT, LPA, and smear microscopy cannot differentiate viable from dead bacilli, retreatment cases may be **overdiagnosed.**
- FDA staining can prevent **unnecessary exposure to toxic second-line TB drugs** by identifying patients who do not need retreatment.

Infection Control and Non-Infectiousness Determination

- According to WHO guidelines, **two consecutive negative sputum smears and cultures taken 30 days apart** are required to declare a patient non-infectious.
- However, cultures take weeks to yield results, delaying infection control decisions.
- The **Centers for Disease Control (CDC) recommends using two consecutive negative Xpert MTB/RIF assays** to determine non-infectiousness.
- FDA staining offers a **faster, cost-effective alternative** to culture-based methods for evaluating infectiousness, especially in resource-limited settings.

FDA Staining as a Replacement for Sputum Culture

- While MGIT liquid culture remains the gold standard for assessing bacterial viability, it is **expensive and time-consuming** (weeks to months for results).
- FDA staining provides a **same-day alternative** for identifying non-viable bacilli in high-burden settings.
- It can be used for **early detection of treatment failure in DR-TB cases.**

Integration into National TB Elimination Programme (NTEP)

- **High-workload DMCs under NTEP** are equipped with WHO-recommended LED fluorescent microscopes.
- Laboratory Technicians (LTs) can be trained to perform FDA staining alongside existing microscopy techniques.

- Using FDA staining in **NTEP laboratories** can help identify patients needing urgent Drug Susceptibility Testing (DST).

Feasibility in Peripheral Laboratories

- **Reagents for FDA staining** are affordable and available at prices similar to ZN and fluorescent staining.
- **Minimal expertise is required** for interpretation, making it suitable for peripheral health centers.
- Standardized protocols can ensure reproducibility and accuracy in **high-burden TB settings.**

Limitations of FDA Staining

While FDA staining offers significant advantages, it has certain limitations:

- **Short Fluorescence Duration:** Fluorescence fades quickly; smears must be examined immediately.
- **Storage Constraints:** The stock solution must be frozen at **-20°C,** and the working solution must be freshly prepared daily.
- **Lack of Standardized Cutoff Values:** Further studies are required to define **quantitative cutoffs** for bacterial viability.
- **Limited Validation in DR-TB:** More research is needed to compare FDA staining with newer molecular methods for **drug resistance detection.**

Conclusion

FDA staining represents a **major advancement in TB diagnostics,** offering a simple, rapid, and cost-effective method to assess bacterial viability in sputum samples. It has the potential to:

- **Improve treatment monitoring** by differentiating between live and dead bacilli.
- **Reduce overdiagnosis** in retreatment cases.
- **Serve as an alternative to MGIT culture** for evaluating drug resistance and non-infectiousness.

By integrating FDA staining into **peripheral laboratories and National TB Programs,** resource-limited settings can benefit from **faster and more accurate TB diagnosis, better treatment decisions, and improved infection control measures.**

Future Prospects in Microscopy-Based TB Diagnosis

While microscopy continues to be an important diagnostic tool, advancements in molecular diagnostics and automated microscopy hold promise for improving sensitivity and specificity. Innovations such as digital image analysis and AI-assisted microscopy are emerging trends that may further revolutionize TB diagnosis in the near future.

20. Culture-Based Diagnostics

Importance of Mycobacterial Culture in TB Diagnosis

Mycobacterial culture remains the gold standard for tuberculosis (TB) diagnosis due to its superior sensitivity compared to microscopy. Unlike smear-based tests, cultures can detect as few as 10 bacilli per milliliter, making them crucial for diagnosing paucibacillary and extrapulmonary TB. Additionally, culture allows for drug susceptibility testing (DST), essential for managing drug-resistant TB cases. Culture methods are also vital for epidemiological studies, surveillance of TB transmission, and identifying outbreaks.

Culture-based methods play a crucial role in diagnosing TB in immunocompromised patients, such as those with HIV/AIDS, in whom traditional smear microscopy may fail due to a low bacterial load. Furthermore, extrapulmonary TB, which affects organs other than the lungs, often requires culture for accurate diagnosis, as smear microscopy and molecular tests may not be as sensitive in these cases.

Solid Culture Methods

Solid culture media have been traditionally used for isolating Mycobacterium tuberculosis. They provide reliable results but require extended incubation times. Solid culture remains valuable in low-resource settings due to its cost-effectiveness and ability to provide drug susceptibility testing.

Löwenstein-Jensen (LJ) Medium

- LJ medium is an egg-based medium commonly used for MTB isolation.
- Contains malachite green to suppress the growth of contaminants.
- MTB colonies appear rough, buff-colored, and slow-growing, taking approximately 4-8 weeks for visible growth.
- Preferred in resource-limited settings due to its simplicity and cost-effectiveness.
- Used for primary isolation and drug susceptibility testing, particularly in developing countries.
- Requires a CO_2-enriched environment for optimal growth, and contamination remains a challenge.

Middlebrook 7H10 and 7H11 Media

- These agar-based synthetic media support faster MTB growth compared to LJ medium.

- Transparent, allowing easier observation of colony morphology.
- Typically used in research and high-throughput laboratories.
- Middlebrook 7H11 contains casein hydrolysate to promote growth.
- Allows for better differentiation between MTB and non-tuberculous mycobacteria (NTM).

Turnaround Time and Colony Morphology Interpretation

- Growth on solid media can take several weeks, leading to delayed diagnosis.
- Colony morphology helps differentiate MTB from non-tuberculous mycobacteria (NTM).
- MTB colonies are rough, dry, and buff-colored, whereas NTM colonies may be pigmented.
- The delayed turnaround time is a significant drawback, necessitating faster culture methods.

5.4.3 Liquid Culture Methods

Liquid culture systems have revolutionized TB diagnostics by reducing turnaround times and increasing sensitivity. These systems enhance MTB recovery rates, particularly for paucibacillary and extrapulmonary cases.

Mycobacteria Growth Indicator Tube (MGIT) System

- MGIT 960 is a fully automated, fluorescence-based culture system.
- Detects MTB growth within 7-14 days, significantly faster than solid culture.
- Contains oxygen-sensitive fluorescence indicators that signal bacterial growth.
- Recommended by the WHO for TB detection and DST.
- More sensitive than solid culture, but prone to contamination if not handled properly.

BACTEC 460 Radiometric System

- Older radiometric system that detects MTB growth based on the release of radioactive carbon dioxide.
- High sensitivity but requires handling of radioactive materials, limiting its use.
- Has been largely replaced by newer, non-radiometric methods due to biosafety concerns.

BACTEC 9000 MB and BacT/Alert MB Systems

- Non-radiometric liquid culture systems that use colorimetric sensors for detecting MTB growth.
- Safer and environmentally friendly alternatives to radiometric methods.
- Faster than solid culture and ideal for high-throughput diagnostic laboratories.
- Automated systems reduce manual workload and improve consistency in results.

Automated Culture Systems

Automated systems have improved the efficiency of TB diagnostics by providing faster and more accurate results. These systems reduce human error, increase throughput, and enhance biosafety.

Advantages in Drug Susceptibility Testing (DST)

- Automated liquid culture systems allow for rapid DST.
- Essential for detecting multidrug-resistant (MDR) and extensively drug-resistant (XDR) TB.
- WHO recommends liquid culture DST as the reference standard for phenotypic drug resistance testing.
- Faster turnaround times allow for early initiation of appropriate TB treatment.
- Provides quantitative growth data, aiding in resistance level determination.

WHO Recommendations on Culture-Based Methods

- Liquid culture is the preferred method in high-burden and resource-equipped settings.
- Solid culture remains relevant for confirmatory testing and epidemiological studies.
- Biosafety level 3 (BSL-3) laboratory facilities are required for handling cultures.
- Laboratories must follow strict quality control and contamination prevention protocols.

Sample Decontamination and Processing for Culture

Mycobacterial culture requires decontamination of samples to prevent contamination from other bacteria. Various methods are used to optimize MTB recovery while minimizing overgrowth by other microorganisms.

- **Sodium hydroxide (NaOH) method:** Decontaminates and liquefies sputum before inoculation. Excessive decontamination can kill MTB, reducing sensitivity.
- **NALC-NaOH method:** Uses N-acetyl-L-cysteine (NALC) as a mucolytic agent to improve MTB recovery. Considered a superior method for preserving viable bacilli.
- **Centrifugation and concentration:** Enhances MTB detection by concentrating bacilli from clinical specimens. Essential for samples with low bacterial loads, such as CSF and pleural fluid.
- **Use of antibiotics (e.g., PANTA):** Some liquid culture systems use antibiotic mixtures to suppress non-mycobacterial contaminants.

Future Directions in Culture-Based Diagnostics

The future of culture-based TB diagnostics lies in improving speed, accuracy, and biosafety.

- Development of faster, non-invasive culture techniques to reduce diagnosis time.
- Use of AI-based image analysis for automated colony detection and interpretation.
- Integration of genotypic and phenotypic testing for comprehensive MTB identification.
- Enhancement of biosafety measures to reduce culture-related infections and improve laboratory safety.
- Molecular culture confirmation methods to rapidly differentiate MTB from non-tuberculous mycobacteria.
- Research into portable culture systems for field-based diagnostics in remote locations.

Conclusion

Culture-based TB diagnosis remains a cornerstone of mycobacteriology. While liquid culture offers faster results and better sensitivity, solid media continue to play a critical role, especially in resource-limited settings. Advancements in automation, AI-driven culture interpretation, and biosafety measures are expected to further enhance the diagnostic capabilities for TB in the coming years. Strengthening laboratory infrastructure and ensuring adherence to biosafety protocols will be crucial for optimizing culture-based TB diagnostics worldwide.

21. Molecular Diagnostics

Nucleic Acid Amplification Tests (NAATs)

Nucleic Acid Amplification Tests (NAATs) represent a groundbreaking advancement in the diagnosis of tuberculosis (TB). These tests offer a rapid, highly sensitive, and specific means of detecting Mycobacterium tuberculosis (MTB) DNA or RNA, significantly reducing diagnostic turnaround time from weeks to mere hours. The WHO has strongly recommended NAATs, particularly in settings with a high burden of multidrug-resistant tuberculosis (MDR-TB), as these tests play a crucial role in early detection and treatment initiation.

GeneXpert MTB/RIF & GeneXpert Ultra

- **Principle:** GeneXpert is a real-time polymerase chain reaction (PCR)-based diagnostic tool that amplifies MTB DNA and simultaneously detects rifampicin resistance by targeting the rpoB gene.
- **Procedure:**
    - Sample processing: The sample is mixed with a lysis buffer to deactivate infectious organisms and release MTB DNA.
    - Cartridge-based amplification: The processed sample is loaded into a self-contained GeneXpert cartridge pre-filled with all necessary PCR reagents.
    - Automated analysis: The GeneXpert system amplifies the target MTB DNA sequences and detects rifampicin resistance mutations within approximately two hours.
- **Detection Limits:**
    - GeneXpert MTB/RIF: Detects MTB at 131 CFU/mL.
    - GeneXpert Ultra: Offers improved sensitivity, detecting as few as 16 CFU/mL, making it more effective for paucibacillary and extrapulmonary TB.
- **Interpretation:**
    - MTB Detected: Positive result with or without rifampicin resistance.
    - MTB Not Detected: Negative result, though clinical correlation is necessary for final diagnosis.
    - Rifampicin Resistance Detected: Suggestive of MDR-TB, requiring confirmation through additional drug susceptibility testing (DST).
- **Clinical Significance of Rifampicin Resistance Detection:**
    - Rifampicin resistance is a strong predictor of MDR-TB.
    - WHO recommends second-line DST for patients with rifampicin resistance.

- Early detection allows appropriate treatment initiation, reducing TB transmission.

Line Probe Assay (LPA)

- **Principle:** Genotypic DST that detects MTB and its resistance to first-line and second-line anti-TB drugs by hybridization of amplified DNA to specific probes.
- **Types of LPAs:**
    - **Hain Test (MTBDRplus, MTBDRsl):**
        - MTBDRplus detects resistance to rifampicin and isoniazid.
        - MTBDRsl identifies resistance to fluoroquinolones and injectable second-line drugs.
    - **Newer Advancements:**
        - Expanded detection panels for pyrazinamide resistance.
        - Improved sensitivity for extrapulmonary TB samples.
- **Advantages:**
    - Rapid turnaround time (24-48 hours).
    - Detects MDR-TB and extensively drug-resistant TB (XDR-TB).
- **Limitations:**
    - Requires skilled personnel and well-equipped molecular laboratories.
    - Cannot detect novel mutations or rare resistance patterns.

Loop-Mediated Isothermal Amplification (LAMP)

- **Principle:** LAMP uses a set of primers and Bst polymerase to amplify MTB DNA at a constant temperature (60-65°C), eliminating the need for thermal cycling.
- **Advantages in Resource-Limited Settings:**
    - Does not require sophisticated thermal cyclers.
    - Rapid detection (30-60 minutes) with high specificity.
    - Visual detection through color change, eliminating the need for complex instrumentation.
    - Can be implemented at the point of care (POC) in low-resource settings.
- **Limitations:**
    - Lower sensitivity for paucibacillary TB.
    - Contamination risks due to high amplification efficiency.

Whole-Genome Sequencing (WGS) and Next-Generation Sequencing (NGS)

Role in TB Epidemiology, Resistance Prediction, and Strain Typing

- **Epidemiology:**
  - WGS enables tracking of TB transmission chains and outbreak investigations.
  - Helps differentiate reactivation from reinfection in recurrent TB cases.
- **Resistance Prediction:**
  - Identifies known and novel mutations associated with drug resistance.
  - Predicts resistance profiles for multiple drugs in a single assay, reducing reliance on phenotypic DST.
- **Strain Typing:**
  - Differentiates MTB strains to study transmission dynamics.
  - Used for surveillance of MDR-TB and XDR-TB strains.
- **Challenges:**
  - High cost and infrastructure requirements.
  - Data interpretation requires bioinformatics expertise.
  - Not yet widely available in resource-limited settings.

Other PCR-Based Methods

Real-Time PCR and Conventional PCR Techniques

- **Real-Time PCR:**
  - Quantitative PCR (qPCR) detects MTB DNA in real-time, providing rapid and specific detection.
  - Used in high-throughput laboratories for TB screening and research.
  - More sensitive than conventional PCR but requires sophisticated instruments.
- **Conventional PCR:**
  - Uses gel electrophoresis for detection.
  - Slower and less sensitive than real-time PCR but still useful in low-resource settings.
  - Requires post-PCR processing, increasing the risk of contamination.

Xpert XDR-TB: Detecting Pre-XDR and XDR Strains

- **Principle:**
    - Expands upon GeneXpert technology to detect resistance beyond rifampicin.
    - Targets resistance mutations in fluoroquinolones, second-line injectables, and bedaquiline.
- **Significance:**
    - Identifies pre-XDR-TB (resistant to rifampicin and fluoroquinolones) and XDR-TB (additionally resistant to second-line injectables and newer drugs).
    - Guides clinicians in selecting appropriate treatment regimens.
- **Limitations:**
    - Higher cost compared to standard GeneXpert MTB/RIF.
    - Requires validation in different clinical settings.

Conclusion

Molecular diagnostics have transformed TB detection by providing rapid, sensitive, and specific results. GeneXpert, LPA, LAMP, and WGS are critical tools in modern TB diagnostics, aiding in early detection and resistance profiling. While molecular methods offer significant advantages, challenges remain, including cost, infrastructure, and skilled personnel requirements. Future advancements in automation, miniaturization, and bioinformatics-driven analysis are expected to further enhance the role of molecular diagnostics in TB control.

22. Immunodiagnostic Approaches

Tuberculin Skin Test (TST, Mantoux Test)

Historical Background and Evolution

The Tuberculin Skin Test (TST), also known as the Mantoux test, was developed by Charles Mantoux in the early 20th century as an improvement over previous tuberculin tests. The test has remained an important diagnostic tool in tuberculosis (TB) screening programs worldwide. Despite the advent of modern diagnostic tools, TST continues to be widely used, particularly in resource-limited settings.

Mechanism

TST is based on the delayed-type hypersensitivity (DTH) reaction, which is a cell-mediated immune response triggered by the injection of purified protein derivative (PPD). The reaction occurs due to prior sensitization to Mycobacterium tuberculosis (MTB) antigens, either from a natural infection or BCG vaccination.

- PPD is injected intradermally, stimulating memory T-cells in previously infected individuals.
- Activated T-cells release cytokines, leading to localized induration at the injection site.
- The test reflects immune memory but cannot differentiate between latent TB infection (LTBI) and active TB disease.

Procedure

1. **Preparation:** A standard dose of 0.1 mL PPD solution containing 5 Tuberculin Units (TU) is prepared.
2. **Injection:** Using a 27-gauge needle, the solution is injected intradermally into the volar aspect of the forearm, producing a visible wheal (6-10 mm).
3. **Reading the Result:** Induration (not erythema) is measured in millimeters after 48-72 hours.
4. **Interpretation:**
    - ≥5 mm: Considered positive in HIV-positive individuals, recent TB contacts, and immunosuppressed patients.
    - ≥10 mm: Positive in recent immigrants from TB-endemic regions, healthcare workers, and children under 4 years.
    - ≥15 mm: Positive in individuals without known TB risk factors.

Factors Affecting TST Results

- **False Positives:** Caused by prior **BCG vaccination** or **infection with nontuberculous mycobacteria.**
- **False Negatives:** Occur in **immunocompromised individuals, recent TB infection, young children,** or **overwhelming TB disease.**
- **Booster Effect:** Repeated TSTs in individuals with past TB exposure can lead to an increased reaction due to immune memory.

Interferon-Gamma Release Assays (IGRAs)

Introduction to IGRAs

Interferon-Gamma Release Assays (IGRAs) represent a major advancement in TB diagnostics by measuring IFN-γ production from T-cells in response to MTB-specific antigens. Unlike TST, IGRAs do not cross-react with BCG and most nontuberculous mycobacteria, improving specificity.

Types of IGRAs

QuantiFERON-TB Gold Plus (QFT-Plus)

- Uses **whole blood** to measure IFN-γ production in response to MTB-specific antigens.
- Requires **four tubes**: Nil (negative control), TB1 (CD4+ response), TB2 (CD4+ and CD8+ response), Mitogen (positive control).
- A positive result suggests MTB infection but does not distinguish between latent and active TB.
- Sensitivity: 85-90%, Specificity: ~98%.

T-SPOT.TB Test

- Uses **peripheral blood mononuclear cells (PBMCs)** instead of whole blood.
- ELISPOT assay detects IFN-γ -secreting T-cells.
- More sensitive in immunocompromised patients compared to QFT-Plus.
- Less affected by factors like low lymphocyte count.

Comparative Sensitivity and Specificity vs. TST

- IGRAs are **more specific** than TST as they do not cross-react with BCG.
- IGRAs have **higher sensitivity** in immunosuppressed patients.
- TST remains useful in **high-risk populations** due to lower cost.
- IGRAs do not require a return visit for result interpretation, unlike TST.

Applications in Latent TB Infection (LTBI) Diagnosis

- Preferred in **BCG-vaccinated individuals** to avoid false positives.
- Used in **healthcare workers and contacts of active TB patients.**
- Recommended for **immunosuppressed individuals,** including transplant candidates and HIV-positive patients.
- Plays a key role in **TB elimination strategies** by identifying LTBI cases for preventive treatment.

Advantages of IGRAs Over TST

- Single visit test; no need for patient return.
- No boosting phenomenon.
- Not affected by BCG vaccination.
- More precise quantification of immune response.

Most recent Skin Test: C-Tb (Cytokine-Tuberculosis) Test

The **C-Tb (Cytokine-Tuberculosis) Test** is a **next-generation skin test** developed as a more specific alternative to the **Mantoux (Tuberculin Skin Test - TST)** for detecting **latent tuberculosis infection (LTBI).** It is designed to overcome the limitations of the Mantoux test, particularly its cross-reactivity with the **BCG vaccine** and **non-tuberculous mycobacteria (NTM).**

Key Features of the C-Tb Test

Uses Specific TB Antigens

- Unlike Mantoux, which uses **purified protein derivative (PPD)**, C-Tb contains:
  - **ESAT-6 (Early Secretory Antigenic Target-6)**
  - **CFP-10 (Culture Filtrate Protein-10)**
- These antigens are unique to *Mycobacterium tuberculosis* and are **not present in BCG vaccine strains** or most NTMs, making the test more **specific for TB infection.**

Mechanism

- Works **similarly to the Mantoux test,** where a **small amount of antigen is injected intradermally** (under the skin).
- If the person has been exposed to *M. tuberculosis*, their immune system produces a **localized skin reaction** (induration), which is measured 48-72 hours later.

Advantages Over the Mantoux Test

- **More specific:** Reduces false positives in BCG-vaccinated individuals.
- **Comparable sensitivity** to both **TST** and **Interferon-Gamma Release Assays (IGRAs)** like **QuantiFERON-TB Gold Plus.**
- **Easier to administer:** Works like Mantoux but with better specificity.
- **Cost-effective alternative** to blood-based tests like IGRA.

Advantages of the C-Tb Test

✓ **More Specific Than Mantoux (TST) -** Uses **ESAT-6 and CFP-10,** which are absent in **BCG and most non-tuberculous mycobacteria (NTM), reducing false positives** in vaccinated individuals.

✓ **Easier and Cheaper Than IGRA -** Unlike **IGRAs (QuantiFERON & T-SPOT.TB),** C-Tb does **not** require **specialized lab equipment, blood collection, or processing,** making it **cost-effective** for low-resource settings.

✓ **Comparable Sensitivity to IGRA -** Sensitivity of **85-90%** (higher than Mantoux and close to IGRA tests).

✓ **Compatible with Existing TB Screening Programs -** Since it works similarly to Mantoux (TST), **healthcare workers do not need new training.**

Limitations of the C-Tb Test

✗ **Still Requires Follow-Up Visit (Like Mantoux) -** Patients must **return in 48-72 hours** for measurement of the induration (raised skin reaction).

✗ **Potential Cross-Reactivity with Some Environmental Mycobacteria -** Although rare, some non-tuberculous mycobacteria (NTM) **may cause false positives.**

✗ **Not Yet Widely Available -** Currently undergoing trials but **not yet WHO-approved for global TB screening.**

Clinical Trials & Current Status

- **Developed by: Statens Serum Institut (SSI), Denmark).**
- **Clinical trials:**

- Show **comparable performance to IGRA** and **better specificity than Mantoux.**
- Effective in **BCG-vaccinated individuals** and **HIV-positive patients.**

- **Regulatory approvals:**
  - Awaiting **WHO endorsement** for widespread use in TB screening programs.

Future of the C-Tb Test

The **C-Tb test is a strong candidate to replace the Mantoux test** due to its **higher specificity, ease of use, and affordability compared to IGRA.** If approved by the **WHO and national TB programs,** it could become the **new standard for TB screening worldwide.**

Global Guidelines and Recommendations

WHO Recommendations

- WHO recommends IGRAs for latent TB infection diagnosis in **high-income settings** but continues to endorse TST in **resource-limited regions.**
- IGRAs are particularly useful in **low-TB prevalence settings** where false-positive TST results are more common.
- Routine use of IGRAs for **active TB diagnosis** is not recommended due to poor differentiation between active and latent TB.

CDC Guidelines

- IGRAs preferred over TST in individuals with **BCG vaccination history.**
- Healthcare workers and close contacts should be screened using IGRAs or TST based on feasibility and setting.
- In **HIV-infected patients,** IGRAs should be used cautiously as immune suppression can reduce IFN-γ response.

European Guidelines

- The European Centre for Disease Prevention and Control (ECDC) advocates for **dual testing** (TST + IGRA) in high-risk populations to improve sensitivity.
- IGRAs are widely implemented in **occupational health screenings.**

Future Directions in Immunodiagnostics

Emerging Biomarkers

- Research is underway to identify novel biomarkers, such as TNF-α , IP-10, and IL-2, to improve TB diagnostic accuracy.
- Multiplex assays combining IGRA with additional immune markers may enhance sensitivity.

Next-Generation IGRA Technologies

- Development of point-of-care IGRA tests to enable rapid TB screening.
- High-throughput IGRA platforms to improve large-scale screening efficiency.

Integration with Digital Health Technologies

- Use of AI-driven analysis for IGRA and TST interpretation.
- Mobile health applications to track and manage LTBI cases.

Conclusion

Immunodiagnostic approaches remain crucial for TB screening and detection. While the Mantoux test is still widely used, IGRAs offer superior specificity and practicality. Future research and advancements aim to further refine these diagnostic tools, ultimately aiding in global TB control efforts.

23. Biomarkers and Serological Tests

Serodiagnostic Tests for TB (Not WHO Recommended)

Introduction

Serological tests for tuberculosis (TB) have long been explored as potential diagnostic tools due to their ability to detect Mycobacterium tuberculosis (MTB)-specific antibodies or antigens in body fluids. These tests offer the promise of rapid and easy-to-perform diagnostics but have not gained widespread acceptance due to limitations in accuracy. In 2011, the World Health Organization (WHO) issued a strong recommendation against the use of commercial serodiagnostic tests for active TB diagnosis due to their poor sensitivity and specificity. However, research into novel serological approaches continues in an effort to develop more reliable methods.

The fundamental premise of serodiagnostic tests lies in detecting an immune response against MTB rather than the pathogen itself. These tests typically employ enzyme-linked immunosorbent assay (ELISA), lateral flow immunoassays, or immunoblots to identify circulating antibodies or MTB antigens. However, given the complex immunopathology of TB, these approaches have faced significant challenges.

Antibody-Based Assays

Serological TB tests rely on identifying host antibodies generated against MTB antigens. The most commonly targeted antigens include:

- **38-kDa antigen** – Found in the cell wall of MTB and implicated in immune recognition.
- **Ag85 complex** – A mycolyltransferase complex essential for MTB virulence.
- **Lipoarabinomannan (LAM)** – A component of the MTB cell wall detectable in body fluids.
- **ESAT-6 and CFP-10** – Secreted proteins associated with virulence and immune response activation.

Despite the theoretical potential of these markers, antibody-based assays have performed poorly in clinical settings. Their primary drawbacks include:

- **Variability in immune response:** Antibody production is inconsistent among TB patients, particularly those who are immunocompromised or co-infected with HIV.

- **Inability to distinguish between active and past infections:** The presence of antibodies does not indicate ongoing infection, making these tests unsuitable for active TB diagnosis.
- **High rates of false positives:** Cross-reactivity with non-tuberculous mycobacteria (NTM) leads to misleading results.
- **Poor sensitivity in extrapulmonary and latent TB cases:** Many individuals do not mount a robust humoral response, particularly in non-pulmonary TB.

Given these challenges, WHO has strongly discouraged the use of antibody-based serological tests for TB. However, efforts continue to improve their accuracy through novel antigen combinations and high-throughput assay platforms.

Clinical Applications and Limitations

Despite their shortcomings, serodiagnostic tests have been used in certain settings, particularly in private-sector laboratories in low-income countries. Their rapid turnaround time and ease of use have made them attractive in areas where conventional diagnostics are unavailable. However, their lack of reliability has resulted in WHO advocating for their discontinuation in routine clinical use.

Host Biomarker-Based Tests

Cytokine-Based Assays

Host biomarker-based diagnostics aim to detect immune mediators that are differentially expressed in TB infection. Among these, cytokine-based assays have garnered significant attention. Cytokines are signaling proteins released by immune cells in response to infection, and their profiles can provide insights into TB pathogenesis.

- **Key Biomarkers in TB Diagnosis:**
  - **Interferon-gamma (IFN-γ):** The basis of Interferon-Gamma Release Assays (IGRAs) used for latent TB detection.
  - **Interleukin-2 (IL-2):** Associated with an active immune response and useful in distinguishing latent from active TB.
  - **Interleukin-6 (IL-6):** Plays a role in inflammation and TB disease severity.
  - **IP-10 (Interferon-gamma inducible protein 10):** Shows promise in enhancing diagnostic sensitivity, especially in pediatric and HIV-positive TB cases.
  - **Tumor Necrosis Factor-alpha (TNF-α):** A key inflammatory cytokine involved in TB immune response.

Cytokine-based assays, particularly those combining multiple markers, hold promise for early and accurate TB detection. However, these tests are not yet widely implemented due to cost and infrastructure limitations.

Use of Transcriptomics in TB Diagnosis

Transcriptomics involves studying gene expression profiles to identify TB-specific signatures. Advances in RNA sequencing (RNA-Seq) have facilitated the discovery of gene signatures associated with TB.

- **Key Gene Signatures:**
    - **BATF2 (Basic Leucine Zipper ATF-Like Transcription Factor 2):** Upregulated in active TB patients.
    - **GBP5 (Guanylate-Binding Protein 5):** Involved in immune response against mycobacterial infections.
    - **LINC01128:** A long non-coding RNA associated with TB pathogenesis.

These transcriptomic markers have demonstrated high specificity for TB and may soon complement existing diagnostic methods. However, their clinical adoption is hindered by cost and the need for advanced laboratory infrastructure.

Proteomics and Metabolomics in TB Diagnosis

Proteomics and metabolomics aim to identify MTB-specific proteins and metabolites in clinical samples.

- **Proteomic Biomarkers:**
    - **ESAT-6 and CFP-10:** Secreted proteins detected in active TB cases.
    - **LAM:** Used in rapid point-of-care tests, particularly in HIV-associated TB.
- **Metabolomic Biomarkers:**
    - MTB infection alters host lipid metabolism, leading to the identification of specific lipid biomarkers.
    - Urinary and blood-based metabolite profiles are being explored for non-invasive TB detection.

Future Directions in Biomarker-Based TB Diagnostics

- **Development of Multiplex Biomarker Panels:**
    - Combining cytokines, transcriptomic, and proteomic markers to improve diagnostic accuracy.
    - AI-driven diagnostic algorithms for real-time TB detection.

- **Point-of-Care Biomarker Tests:**
  - Development of portable, low-cost biomarker assays for use in resource-limited settings.
  - Exploration of breath-based and urine-based diagnostics for non-invasive TB testing.
- **Integration with Digital Health Technologies:**
  - Smartphone-based diagnostic platforms for real-time TB surveillance.
  - Data sharing for epidemiological monitoring and TB control programs.

Conclusion

Serodiagnostic tests for TB have been largely discredited due to their poor performance, but research into host biomarker-based diagnostics is promising. Cytokine assays, transcriptomics, proteomics, and metabolomics are emerging as potential alternatives to conventional methods. The integration of these novel approaches with digital health solutions could transform TB diagnostics in the near future, making them more accessible and accurate. Continued investment in biomarker research and validation studies is crucial for integrating these advancements into routine clinical practice.

24. Radiological and Imaging Techniques in TB Diagnosis

Chest X-Ray (CXR) and Scoring Systems

Introduction

Chest X-ray (CXR) is one of the most widely used diagnostic tools in tuberculosis (TB) diagnosis, particularly for screening and identifying pulmonary TB. While CXR is not definitive for TB confirmation, it plays a crucial role in early detection, particularly in resource-limited settings where molecular and culture-based tests are not readily available. The interpretation of CXR findings requires clinical correlation, and AI-assisted tools are now being explored to enhance accuracy.

Features Suggestive of Active vs. Healed TB

- **Active Pulmonary TB:**
    - Patchy or confluent opacities, often in the upper lobes
    - Cavitations (indicative of necrotizing lesions)
    - Consolidation with tree-in-bud appearance
    - Miliary pattern (small nodular opacities throughout the lung fields)
    - Pleural effusion (can indicate extrapulmonary involvement)
- **Healed or Latent TB:**
    - Fibrotic scarring and volume loss
    - Calcified granulomas (Ghon focus, Ranke complex)
    - Pleural thickening
    - Bronchiectasis and architectural distortion

WHO-Endorsed AI-Assisted CXR Interpretation

With advancements in artificial intelligence, WHO has endorsed AI-assisted CXR interpretation as a tool to improve TB detection, particularly in mass screening programs. AI algorithms are trained to detect abnormalities suggestive of TB, reducing inter-observer variability and improving sensitivity in high-burden settings.

Computed Tomography (CT) and Magnetic Resonance Imaging (MRI)

CT Scan in TB Diagnosis

CT imaging provides detailed visualization of lung structures and is particularly useful in cases where CXR findings are inconclusive. It plays a crucial role in diagnosing both pulmonary and extrapulmonary TB.

- **Findings in Pulmonary TB:**
    - Centrilobular nodules and tree-in-bud appearance
    - Cavitary lesions with thickened walls
    - Ground-glass opacities (suggestive of early infection or immune response)
    - Bronchogenic dissemination patterns
- **Findings in Extrapulmonary TB:**
    - **Mediastinal TB:** Enlarged lymph nodes with necrotic centers
    - **Abdominal TB:** Thickened bowel loops, mesenteric lymphadenopathy, ascites
    - **Spinal TB (Pott's disease):** Vertebral destruction, paravertebral abscesses, spinal cord compression

MRI in TB Diagnosis

MRI is particularly useful in assessing TB involvement in soft tissues, the central nervous system, and bones.

- **Neuro-TB (TB meningitis, tuberculomas):**
    - Basal meningeal enhancement
    - Hydrocephalus and infarctions
    - Ring-enhancing lesions
- **Spinal TB:**
    - Vertebral body collapse (Gibbus deformity)
    - Epidural abscess formation
    - Cord compression signs
- **Musculoskeletal TB:**
    - Joint effusion and synovial thickening
    - Bone erosions in advanced cases

Ultrasound in TB Diagnosis

Ultrasonography is an emerging tool for TB diagnosis, particularly for extrapulmonary TB.

Abdominal TB

- Bowel wall thickening (ileocecal region)
- Mesenteric lymphadenopathy with necrotic centers
- Free or loculated ascitic fluid with septations

Lymph Node TB (Tuberculous Lymphadenitis)

- Enlarged lymph nodes with central necrosis
- Matting of nodes
- Calcifications in chronic cases

Pleural Effusion in TB

- Complex septated effusion (suggestive of TB origin)
- Pleural thickening
- Subdiaphragmatic abscess formation

Positron Emission Tomography (PET-CT) in TB Diagnosis

PET-CT is an advanced imaging modality that provides functional and metabolic insights into TB lesions. It is particularly useful in cases of:

- **Diagnosis of TB when other tests are inconclusive:** PET-CT can differentiate between active TB and non-infectious granulomas.
- **Monitoring Treatment Response:** High FDG uptake indicates active infection, while resolution of uptake correlates with effective treatment.
- **Identifying Disseminated TB:** Helps locate TB involvement in multiple organs, particularly in immunocompromised patients.

Conclusion

Radiological and imaging techniques are integral to TB diagnosis, particularly in cases where microbiological confirmation is challenging. From conventional CXR to advanced PET-CT, imaging modalities enhance early detection, assess disease burden, and monitor treatment response. The integration of AI and emerging technologies holds promise for improving TB diagnostic accuracy and accessibility globally.

25. Drug Susceptibility Testing (DST)

Introduction to Drug Susceptibility Testing (DST)

Drug susceptibility testing (DST) is crucial in the management of tuberculosis (TB) to determine resistance to first-line and second-line anti-TB drugs. With the rise of multidrug-resistant (MDR-TB) and extensively drug-resistant TB (XDR-TB), DST plays a pivotal role in guiding appropriate treatment regimens and preventing the spread of resistant strains.

Phenotypic DST

Proportion Method

The proportion method is a conventional and widely accepted phenotypic DST technique.

- **Principle:** Measures the proportion of mycobacterial population resistant to a specific drug by comparing colony counts on drug-containing and drug-free media.
- **Procedure:**
    - Inoculation of Mycobacterium tuberculosis on Löwenstein-Jensen or Middlebrook agar with and without drugs.
    - Incubation at 37°C for 3-4 weeks.
    - Comparison of growth on control and drug-containing media to determine resistance.
- **Limitations:**
    - Long turnaround time (up to 6 weeks).
    - Requires biosafety level 3 (BSL-3) facilities.

MGIT-Based DST

Mycobacteria Growth Indicator Tube (MGIT) is a liquid culture-based phenotypic DST.

- **Principle:** Fluorescence-based detection of mycobacterial growth in the presence of drugs.
- **Procedure:**
    - Inoculation of TB bacteria into MGIT tubes with and without anti-TB drugs.
    - Automated monitoring of fluorescence changes indicating bacterial growth.

  - Results are interpreted based on time to positivity.
- **Advantages:**
  - Faster results (7-14 days).
  - Higher sensitivity than solid media.
- **Limitations:**
  - Risk of contamination.
  - Requires specialized equipment (BACTEC MGIT 960 system).

Genotypic DST

Genotypic DST detects specific mutations associated with drug resistance using molecular techniques.

Rifampicin Resistance (rpoB Mutations)

- Rifampicin resistance is mainly due to mutations in the rpoB gene.
- **Genotypic detection methods:**
  - GeneXpert MTB/RIF assay.
  - Line probe assays (LPA) detecting rpoB mutations.
  - Whole-genome sequencing (WGS) for detailed resistance profiling.
- **Clinical significance:**
  - Rifampicin resistance often indicates MDR-TB.
  - Requires additional testing for isoniazid resistance.

Isoniazid Resistance (katG and inhA Mutations)

- **katG mutations (e.g., S315T):** High-level isoniazid resistance.
- **inhA promoter mutations:** Low-level resistance, can be overcome by dose adjustments.
- **Genotypic detection:**
  - Line probe assays (MTBDRplus).
  - Real-time PCR and sequencing methods.

Fluoroquinolone Resistance (gyrA and gyrB Mutations)

- Mutations in gyrA and gyrB genes confer resistance to fluoroquinolones like moxifloxacin and levofloxacin.
- **Genotypic detection:**
  - MTBDRsl assay.
  - Whole-genome sequencing.
  - Pyrosequencing.
- **Clinical significance:**

- Fluoroquinolone resistance suggests pre-XDR or XDR-TB.

Second-Line DST Approaches

- **Ethionamide and Prothionamide Resistance:** Detected via inhA mutations.
- **Kanamycin, Amikacin, and Capreomycin Resistance:** Associated with rrs and eis promoter mutations.
- **Bedaquiline and Delamanid Resistance:** Emerging resistance detected by mutations in atpE, fgd1, and ddn genes.

Comparison of Phenotypic and Genotypic DST

Parameter	Phenotypic DST	Genotypic DST
Turnaround Time	2-6 weeks	1-2 days
Detection Method	Growth-based	DNA/RNA mutation detection
Drug Resistance Identified	All drugs tested	Only known resistance-associated mutations
Biosafety Requirement	BSL-3 facility required	BSL-2 facility sufficient
Application	Confirmatory for resistance	Rapid screening tool

WHO Recommendations on DST

- **Rifampicin resistance:** GeneXpert recommended as the initial test.
- **Isoniazid resistance:** LPA or targeted sequencing.
- **Second-line DST:** MTBDRsl assay or WGS.
- **Phenotypic DST confirmation:** Required for inconclusive genotypic results.

Conclusion

Drug susceptibility testing is essential for TB management and resistance surveillance. Phenotypic methods remain the gold standard for DST, but genotypic assays provide rapid results. Advances in molecular diagnostics, including next-generation sequencing, continue to improve the accuracy and speed of DST, enabling better treatment strategies and control measures for TB globally.

26. Diagnosis of Latent TB Infection (LTBI)

Introduction to Latent TB Infection (LTBI)

Latent tuberculosis infection (LTBI) is a crucial component of TB control programs worldwide. Unlike active TB, LTBI is a state in which individuals are infected with *Mycobacterium tuberculosis* but do not show symptoms and cannot transmit the disease. However, they remain at risk of developing active TB, especially if they become immunocompromised. Diagnosing and treating LTBI is essential for controlling TB transmission and achieving TB elimination goals set by the World Health Organization (WHO).

Importance in TB Control Programs

LTBI poses a significant public health challenge, particularly in high-burden and low-resource settings. Effective identification and management of LTBI can:

- Reduce the reservoir of TB infection.
- Prevent progression to active TB, especially in high-risk individuals (e.g., people with HIV, diabetics, and immunosuppressed patients).
- Aid in achieving TB elimination by breaking the chain of transmission.
- Optimize TB control efforts by targeting high-risk populations.

Diagnostic Approaches for LTBI

Since LTBI is asymptomatic, its diagnosis relies on immunological tests that detect the host's immune response to *M. tuberculosis* antigens. These include:

- **Tuberculin Skin Test (TST, Mantoux Test)**
- **Interferon-Gamma Release Assays (IGRAs)**
- **Cy TB Test**

Comparative Performance of TST vs. IGRA

Feature	TST	IGRA
Sensitivity	Moderate	High
Specificity	Low (BCG interference)	High (no BCG interference)
Turnaround Time	48-72 hours	24 hours
Requirement of Follow-up	Yes	No
Suitability in Immunosuppressed Individuals	Less reliable	More reliable

Overview of Latent TB Diagnostic Tests

Feature	C-Tb Test	Mantoux (TST)	QuantiFERON-TB Gold Plus (QFT-Plus)	T-SPOT.TB
Type	Skin Test	Skin Test	Blood Test (IGRA)	Blood Test (IGRA)
Antigens Used	ESAT-6, CFP-10	Purified Protein Derivative (PPD)	ESAT-6, CFP-10	ESAT-6, CFP-10
Affected by BCG?	**No**	**Yes** (False positives in BCG-vaccinated people)	**No**	**No**
False Positives Due to Non-Tuberculous Mycobacteria (NTM)?	**Rare**	**Common**	**Rare**	**Rare**
Time for Results	48-72 hours	48-72 hours	24 hours	24 hours
Lab Infrastructure Required?	No	No	**Yes (Needs specialized lab)**	**Yes (Needs specialized lab)**
Sensitivity	**High (~85-90%)**	Moderate (~70-80%)	**High (~95%)**	**High (~95%)**
Specificity	**High (~90-95%)**	Low (~60-80%)	**Very High (~97-99%)**	**Very High (~97-99%)**
Cost	Moderate	**Low**	**High**	**High**
Use in Low-Resource Settings	**Good (Easy to perform, no lab needed)**	**Good (No lab needed)**	**Difficult (Needs lab setup, costly)**	**Difficult (Needs lab setup, costly)**

Summary: Which Test Should Be Used?

Scenario	Best Test	Reason
BCG-Vaccinated Individuals	**C-Tb or IGRA**	Avoids false positives caused by Mantoux
Low-Cost TB Screening in Rural Areas	**C-Tb or Mantoux**	No lab needed, easy to perform
Fast, Lab-Based Diagnosis Needed	**IGRA (QFT-Plus or T-SPOT.TB)**	High sensitivity & specificity
TB Screening in HIV Patients	**C-Tb or IGRA**	More reliable than Mantoux

Role of Preventive Therapy Based on Diagnostic Findings

Once LTBI is diagnosed, preventive therapy is recommended to reduce the risk of progression to active TB.

- **First-Line Preventive Therapy:**
  - **Isoniazid (INH) for 6-9 months** (Standard therapy).
  - **Rifampicin for 4 months** (Alternative option).
  - **Isoniazid + Rifapentine (once-weekly for 3 months)** (Short-course regimen).
- **Target Populations for Preventive Therapy:**
  - HIV-positive individuals.
  - Household contacts of active TB cases.
  - Patients receiving immunosuppressive therapy (e.g., TNF-α inhibitors).
  - Individuals with diabetes or chronic kidney disease.

Challenges in LTBI Diagnosis and Management

Despite the availability of TST and IGRAs, several challenges persist:

- **Lack of a gold-standard test for LTBI.**
- **High costs and limited availability of IGRAs in resource-limited settings.**
- **Low adherence to preventive therapy due to prolonged treatment duration.**
- **Difficulty in distinguishing true infection from immune sensitization.**

Future Perspectives in LTBI Diagnosis

Recent advances in LTBI diagnostics aim to improve accuracy, accessibility, and predictive value for progression to active TB. Some promising developments include:

- **Next-generation IGRAs:** Improved biomarkers for predicting reactivation risk.
- **Host-derived biomarkers:** Identification of immune signatures indicating LTBI progression.
- **Point-of-care tests:** Rapid, cost-effective tests for use in field settings.

Conclusion

The diagnosis and management of LTBI are essential for global TB control efforts. While TST and IGRAs remain the primary diagnostic tools, new biomarkers and diagnostic approaches hold promise for more accurate detection. Preventive therapy plays a critical role in reducing TB incidence, and ongoing research aims to enhance diagnostic strategies for better LTBI management. Addressing challenges in implementation, cost, and accessibility will be key to achieving global TB elimination goals.

27. Diagnosis of Extrapulmonary TB

Introduction to Extrapulmonary Tuberculosis (EPTB)

Extrapulmonary tuberculosis (EPTB) refers to TB infections occurring outside the lungs, affecting organs such as the central nervous system (CNS), pleura, lymph nodes, abdomen, bones, joints, and the genitourinary system. EPTB accounts for a significant proportion of TB cases, particularly in immunocompromised individuals, including those with HIV/AIDS. The diagnosis of EPTB is often challenging due to the paucibacillary nature of the disease, the need for invasive sampling, and variable clinical presentations. Hence, a combination of microbiological, molecular, immunological, and imaging techniques is essential for accurate diagnosis.

CNS Tuberculosis

CNS TB, including tuberculous meningitis (TBM), tuberculoma, and spinal TB (Pott's disease), is a severe form of TB with high morbidity and mortality.

CSF Analysis in CNS TB

- **Appearance:** CSF is often clear or slightly turbid.
- **Cell Count:** Predominantly lymphocytic pleocytosis (>50 WBCs/μ L).
- **Protein:** Elevated (>100 mg/dL).
- **Glucose:** Low (<40 mg/dL or <50% of plasma glucose).
- **ADA (Adenosine Deaminase):** Raised (>9 IU/L, though less specific than in pleural TB).
- **PCR for *M. tuberculosis*:** Highly specific but variable sensitivity.
- **Culture:** Gold standard but slow (4-8 weeks on solid media, 2 weeks in liquid culture).
- **Imaging:** MRI with contrast reveals meningeal enhancement, hydrocephalus, or tuberculomas.

Pleural Tuberculosis

Pleural TB is one of the most common forms of EPTB, presenting as pleural effusion or empyema.

Diagnostic Tests for Pleural TB

- **Pleural Fluid Analysis:**
  - Lymphocytic predominant pleural effusion.
  - Protein >3.5 g/dL; high LDH (>2/3 serum LDH).

- **ADA (Adenosine Deaminase):** Sensitivity >90% at a cutoff of 40 IU/L.
- **GeneXpert on Pleural Fluid:** Detects *M. tuberculosis* DNA but has moderate sensitivity.
- **Pleural Biopsy:**
    - Histopathology: Granulomatous inflammation.
    - Culture of biopsy specimens enhances diagnostic yield.

Abdominal Tuberculosis

Abdominal TB can involve peritoneum, intestines, lymph nodes, or solid organs like the liver and spleen.

Diagnostic Modalities

- **Fine Needle Aspiration Cytology (FNAC):** For lymph node TB.
- **Ascitic Fluid Analysis:**
    - High protein content and SAAG <1.1 g/dL.
    - ADA >39 IU/L suggests TB.
- **Biopsy:** Laparoscopic biopsy improves diagnostic accuracy.
- **GeneXpert Ultra on Tissue:** Rapid diagnosis with improved sensitivity.

Osteoarticular Tuberculosis

Osteoarticular TB affects the spine (Pott's disease), joints, and long bones, leading to deformities if untreated.

Diagnostic Tests

- **MRI:** Gold standard imaging for spinal TB.
- **CT-Guided Biopsy:** Improves diagnostic yield.
- **Histopathology:** Caseating granulomas confirm TB.
- **Culture and PCR on Bone Tissue:** Essential for definitive diagnosis.

Genitourinary Tuberculosis (GUTB)

GUTB affects kidneys, ureters, bladder, prostate, and reproductive organs.

Diagnostic Tests

- **Urine TB-PCR:** Detects *M. tuberculosis* DNA in early morning urine samples.
- **Mycobacterial Culture:** Gold standard for GUTB diagnosis.
- **IVU (Intravenous Urography):** Shows strictures, hydronephrosis, and calyceal deformities.

- **Ultrasound and CT Scan:** Detect renal involvement.

Miliary Tuberculosis

Miliary TB is a disseminated form of TB characterized by hematogenous spread to multiple organs.

Diagnostic Methods

- **Chest X-ray (CXR):** "Miliary mottling" pattern (numerous small nodules throughout lungs).
- **Blood Culture:** Yields M. *tuberculosis* in disseminated cases.
- **Bone Marrow Aspiration & Culture:** Detects TB in advanced cases.
- **Molecular Tests (GeneXpert Ultra):** High sensitivity in miliary TB diagnosis.

Conclusion

The diagnosis of extrapulmonary TB is complex, requiring a combination of clinical, microbiological, molecular, and imaging techniques. While traditional methods like culture remain the gold standard, rapid diagnostic tests like GeneXpert Ultra and PCR-based methods have significantly improved detection rates. Effective diagnosis and timely treatment are crucial in reducing morbidity and preventing complications associated with EPTB.

28. Advances in TB Diagnostics

AI-Based TB Screening Tools

Artificial intelligence (AI) has revolutionized TB diagnostics, particularly in resource-limited settings where trained radiologists are scarce. AI-driven software for chest X-ray (CXR) interpretation helps in mass TB screening by detecting abnormal lung patterns indicative of TB.

Key AI-Based TB Screening Tools

- **CAD4TB (Computer-Aided Detection for Tuberculosis):** Uses deep learning algorithms to analyze CXR images and provides a risk score.
- **qXR (Qure.ai):** AI model trained on diverse TB datasets for automated TB detection and severity grading.
- **Lunit INSIGHT CXR:** AI-powered diagnostic aid for TB screening approved by WHO.
- **Google's Deep Learning Model:** Developed in collaboration with FIND for high-accuracy TB detection.

AI models improve diagnostic accuracy and reduce human errors, making them valuable in early TB detection. Studies have demonstrated that AI-assisted CXR interpretation can outperform or match radiologists in detecting TB-related abnormalities, making it a crucial tool in high-burden regions.

Point-of-Care TB Diagnostics for Remote Settings

Traditional TB diagnostics require sophisticated lab infrastructure, making them inaccessible in many high-burden areas. Recent advancements in point-of-care (POC) diagnostics have enabled rapid and field-friendly TB testing, helping to detect and treat cases earlier.

POC Diagnostic Tools

- **GeneXpert Omni:** Portable, battery-operated version of GeneXpert, ideal for remote settings.
- **Truenat MTB/RIF:** Chip-based, rapid molecular test providing results in under an hour.
- **LAM (Lipoarabinomannan) Urine Test:** WHO-endorsed for TB detection in HIV-positive patients.
- **TB LAMP (Loop-Mediated Isothermal Amplification):** High-sensitivity molecular test for field use.

Point-of-care diagnostics significantly reduce the time from suspicion to treatment initiation, which is critical in controlling TB transmission. Their application in mobile health units and outreach programs has enhanced TB case-finding, especially among vulnerable populations.

Nanotechnology-Based Rapid Tests

Nanotechnology has introduced innovative diagnostic approaches that enhance the sensitivity and specificity of TB tests, providing more rapid and accurate results compared to conventional techniques.

Nanotechnology in TB Diagnosis

- **Nanoparticle-Based Biosensors:** Detect TB antigens or nucleic acids with high sensitivity.
- **Quantum Dot (QD) Fluorescence Assays:** Enable rapid TB detection through colorimetric analysis.
- **Gold Nanoparticle-Based Lateral Flow Assays:** Provide quick, affordable, and highly specific TB detection.
- **Magnetic Nanoparticles for TB DNA Extraction:** Improve efficiency of molecular diagnostics.

Nanotechnology enables the development of ultra-sensitive assays that can detect TB bacteria even in paucibacillary cases. The use of gold nanoparticles and biosensors in TB diagnostics holds promise for decentralized testing, where laboratory infrastructure is limited.

CRISPR-Based Diagnostics (SHERLOCK, DETECTR)

CRISPR-based diagnostics have emerged as a groundbreaking technology in TB detection, offering rapid, highly specific, and cost-effective solutions that can outperform traditional PCR-based methods.

SHERLOCK (Specific High-Sensitivity Enzymatic Reporter Unlocking)

- Uses CRISPR-Cas13 enzyme to detect TB RNA.
- Provides results within 30 minutes with minimal equipment.
- Highly specific for *M. tuberculosis* DNA.

DETECTR (DNA Endonuclease Targeted CRISPR Trans Reporter)

- Employs Cas12 for detecting TB DNA.
- Fluorescence-based readout improves diagnostic accuracy.

- Potential integration into portable, field-friendly diagnostic kits.

CRISPR-based assays offer rapid and precise TB detection with minimal processing time. They have the potential to be adapted into cost-effective, easy-to-use formats for low-resource settings.

Emerging Technologies in TB Diagnostics

1. **Wearable Biosensors for TB Monitoring:**
    - Devices capable of detecting TB-specific volatile organic compounds (VOCs) in breath samples.
    - Non-invasive and real-time monitoring of TB progression.
2. **Smartphone-Based TB Detection:**
    - Mobile applications integrated with AI to analyze digitized sputum smear images.
    - Real-time connectivity with centralized databases for case reporting and tracking.
3. **Portable Nucleic Acid Testing (NAT) Platforms:**
    - Battery-operated, ultra-rapid NAT devices that can amplify TB DNA in under 15 minutes.
    - Ideal for use in remote clinics and field settings.

Challenges and Future Perspectives

Despite advancements in TB diagnostics, several challenges remain:

- **Cost and accessibility:** Many of the newer technologies are expensive and require further price reduction for widespread implementation.
- **Regulatory approval:** Emerging diagnostics need extensive validation and regulatory approvals before they can be widely adopted.
- **Integration into health systems:** Ensuring that innovative diagnostics fit into existing TB control programs and treatment protocols.

Future advancements in TB diagnostics should focus on affordability, accuracy, and field applicability. Collaborative efforts among researchers, policymakers, and global health organizations will be crucial in achieving the goal of early and universal TB detection.

Conclusion

The landscape of TB diagnostics is rapidly evolving, with AI, nanotechnology, and CRISPR-based methods significantly improving detection rates, turnaround time, and accessibility. These innovations offer hope for better TB control, particularly in high-burden, resource-limited settings. Future research should prioritize the translation of these cutting-edge technologies into widely accessible and cost-effective diagnostic tools for global TB eradication.

SECTION 6

DRUG RESISTANCE AND TREATMENT STRATEGIES

29. Anti-TB Drugs: Mechanism of Action

Tuberculosis (TB) treatment relies on a combination of first-line and second-line drugs that target different aspects of *Mycobacterium tuberculosis* physiology. Understanding their mechanisms of action is critical in managing drug resistance and optimizing therapy.

First-Line Anti-TB Drugs

1. **Isoniazid (INH)**
   - Inhibits mycolic acid synthesis, an essential component of the mycobacterial cell wall.
   - Requires activation by the bacterial catalase-peroxidase enzyme KatG.
2. **Rifampicin (RIF)**
   - Binds to the β-subunit of RNA polymerase, inhibiting transcription.
   - High bactericidal activity against both active and dormant bacilli.
3. **Ethambutol (EMB)**
   - Inhibits arabinosyl transferase, disrupting cell wall biosynthesis.
   - Prevents bacterial proliferation and enhances penetration of other drugs.
4. **Pyrazinamide (PZA)**
   - Converted into pyrazinoic acid (POA), which disrupts membrane potential and fatty acid synthesis.
   - Effective in acidic environments, particularly within granulomas.
5. **Streptomycin (SM)**
   - Binds to the 30S ribosomal subunit, inhibiting protein synthesis.
   - Used mainly in severe or drug-resistant TB cases.

Second-Line and Newer Anti-TB Drugs

1. **Fluoroquinolones (Levofloxacin, Moxifloxacin)**
   - Inhibit DNA gyrase, preventing bacterial DNA replication.
2. **Aminoglycosides (Amikacin, Kanamycin, Capreomycin)**
   - Target bacterial ribosomes, disrupting protein synthesis.
3. **Bedaquiline**
   - Inhibits ATP synthase, leading to bacterial energy depletion.
4. **Delamanid and Pretomanid**
   - Inhibit mycolic acid synthesis and generate reactive nitrogen species.

30. Multidrug-Resistant TB and Extensively Drug-Resistant TB

Drug-resistant TB (DR-TB) poses significant challenges to treatment and public health.

Classification of Drug-Resistant TB

1. **Multidrug-Resistant TB (MDR-TB)**
    - Resistant to at least isoniazid and rifampicin.
2. **Pre-Extensively Drug-Resistant TB (Pre-XDR-TB)**
    - MDR-TB with additional resistance to fluoroquinolones.
3. **Extensively Drug-Resistant TB (XDR-TB)**
    - Resistant to isoniazid, rifampicin, fluoroquinolones, and at least one second-line injectable drug.

Challenges in Managing DR-TB

- **Longer Treatment Duration:** DR-TB regimens last 9-24 months.
- **Higher Toxicity:** Second-line drugs have severe side effects.
- **Lower Cure Rates:** XDR-TB cure rates are significantly lower than drug-sensitive TB.

31. Molecular Basis of Drug Resistance

M. tuberculosis acquires resistance through genetic mutations rather than horizontal gene transfer.

Key Genetic Mutations

1. **Rifampicin Resistance**
    - Mutations in the *rpoB* gene, encoding RNA polymerase.
2. **Isoniazid Resistance**
    - Mutations in *katG* (activates isoniazid) and *inhA* (mycolic acid synthesis target).
3. **Pyrazinamide Resistance**
    - Mutations in *pncA*, affecting conversion to pyrazinoic acid.
4. **Fluoroquinolone Resistance**
    - Mutations in *gyrA* and *gyrB*, affecting DNA gyrase function.

Newer Anti-TB Drugs and Treatment Guidelines

Bedaquiline-Based Regimens

- Shorter, all-oral regimens with bedaquiline have improved DR-TB outcomes.

WHO Guidelines for Drug-Resistant TB

- **MDR-TB Treatment**: Bedaquiline, linezolid, fluoroquinolones.
- **XDR-TB Treatment**: Newer combinations including pretomanid.

Conclusion

Innovative strategies, rapid molecular diagnostics, and novel drug regimens are essential to combat the rising burden of drug-resistant TB.

SECTION 7

TB VACCINES AND PREVENTION

32. BCG Vaccine: Efficacy and Limitations

The Bacillus Calmette-Guérin (BCG) vaccine is the only licensed vaccine for tuberculosis (TB) and has been in use for nearly a century. Despite its widespread use, BCG has variable efficacy, especially in adults.

Efficacy of BCG

1. **Protection in Children:**
   - Provides 70-80% protection against severe forms of TB, such as tuberculous meningitis and miliary TB.
   - Less effective in preventing pulmonary TB in adults.
2. **Variability in Effectiveness:**
   - Protection differs by geographic region; highest efficacy is observed in populations farther from the equator.
   - Environmental mycobacteria exposure may interfere with vaccine efficacy.
   - Genetic and immunological differences in populations may also affect the vaccine's protective effect.
3. **Mechanism of Protection:**
   - Induces a strong Th1 immune response, which is crucial in containing *M. tuberculosis*.
   - Triggers trained immunity, where innate immune cells develop a memory-like response.

Limitations of BCG

1. **Does Not Prevent Primary Infection:**
   - BCG does not completely prevent infection with *Mycobacterium tuberculosis*.
   - Some vaccinated individuals still develop active TB later in life.
2. **Limited Impact on Adult Pulmonary TB:**
   - Its effectiveness in preventing adult pulmonary TB is inconsistent, ranging from 0% to 80% in various studies.
   - The immunity conferred by BCG wanes over time, requiring potential booster doses.
3. **Interference with Tuberculin Skin Test (TST):**
   - Causes false-positive results in TST-based latent TB diagnosis.
   - This creates challenges in distinguishing BCG-vaccinated individuals from those with latent TB infection.
4. **Safety Concerns in Immunocompromised Individuals:**

- BCG is a live attenuated vaccine and can cause disseminated BCG infection in people with HIV/AIDS or severe immunosuppression.

33. New and Emerging TB Vaccines

Given the limitations of BCG, several new vaccine candidates are under investigation.

Types of TB Vaccines in Development

1. **Live Attenuated Vaccines**
   - Genetically modified BCG or M. *tuberculosis* strains designed to enhance immune response.
   - Examples include MTBVAC, a weakened M. *tuberculosis* strain with improved immunogenicity.
2. **Subunit Vaccines**
   - Contain specific antigens (e.g., Ag85, ESAT-6) to stimulate immunity.
   - Typically require adjuvants to enhance immune response.
3. **Viral Vector-Based Vaccines**
   - Use viral vectors (e.g., adenovirus) to deliver TB antigens to the immune system.
   - Example: MVA85A, which was tested as a BCG booster.
4. **mRNA Vaccines**
   - Similar to COVID-19 vaccines, mRNA vaccines for TB are being explored for their ability to induce robust immunity.
   - Advantages include rapid production and strong cellular immunity stimulation.

Promising TB Vaccine Candidates

1. **MTBVAC**
   - A live attenuated M. *tuberculosis* vaccine currently in clinical trials.
   - Expected to provide broader immunity compared to BCG.
2. **M72/AS01E**
   - A subunit vaccine showing promising results in preventing progression from latent to active TB.
   - Demonstrated around 50% efficacy in clinical trials.
3. **VPM1002**
   - A recombinant BCG vaccine with enhanced immunogenicity.
   - Shows potential for use in both newborns and adults as a booster.
4. **DAR-901**
   - Derived from an inactivated non-tuberculous mycobacterium.

- Investigated as a booster vaccine for previously BCG-vaccinated individuals.

34. Infection Control and Preventive Strategies

Beyond vaccination, infection control measures are essential to prevent TB transmission.

TB Infection Control in Healthcare Settings

1. **Administrative Controls**
   - Early diagnosis and isolation of TB cases.
   - Implementation of TB screening programs for healthcare workers.
   - Prompt initiation of treatment to reduce transmission risk.
2. **Environmental Controls**
   - Proper ventilation in healthcare facilities.
   - Use of ultraviolet germicidal irradiation (UVGI) to kill airborne *M. tuberculosis*.
   - High-efficiency particulate air (HEPA) filtration systems in high-risk settings.
3. **Personal Protective Equipment (PPE)**
   - Use of N95 respirators by healthcare workers.
   - Masking of TB patients to reduce transmission.

Community-Level TB Prevention Strategies

1. **Active Case Finding**
   - Screening high-risk populations (e.g., prisoners, people living with HIV) for TB.
   - Use of mobile diagnostic units to reach remote communities.
2. **Treatment of Latent TB Infection (LTBI)**
   - Preventive therapy using isoniazid or rifapentine in individuals with LTBI.
   - New short-course regimens like 3HP (once-weekly isoniazid + rifapentine for 3 months) improve adherence.
3. **Public Awareness and Education**
   - Campaigns to promote early diagnosis and treatment adherence.
   - Community health workers play a crucial role in TB education and stigma reduction.
4. **Improving Nutrition and Living Conditions**
   - Malnutrition and overcrowding increase TB susceptibility.

    - Policies promoting better housing and nutrition can reduce TB transmission.

35. Global TB Vaccination and Prevention Policies

WHO Strategies and Recommendations

- The WHO End TB Strategy aims to reduce TB incidence by 90% and TB mortality by 95% by 2035.
- BCG vaccination remains part of national immunization programs in TB-endemic countries.
- Research and funding efforts are directed toward developing new vaccines and preventive therapies.

Challenges in TB Prevention

- Limited access to new TB vaccines in low-income countries.
- Vaccine hesitancy and misinformation hinder uptake.
- Drug-resistant TB strains require novel prevention and treatment approaches.

Future Directions in TB Prevention

- Integration of AI-based diagnostic tools with TB screening programs.
- Development of next-generation TB vaccines with long-lasting immunity.
- Expansion of preventive therapy programs to high-risk populations.

Conclusion

While BCG remains a cornerstone of TB prevention, novel vaccines and strengthened infection control measures are crucial in achieving TB elimination. Ongoing research into new vaccine candidates offers hope for a more effective and long-lasting solution to TB prevention. The integration of innovative strategies, including AI-assisted diagnostics, nanotechnology-based detection, and improved public health interventions, will be vital in reducing the TB burden globally.

SECTION 8

ADVANCES AND FUTURE DIRECTIONS IN TUBERCULOSIS RESEARCH

36. Whole-Genome Sequencing in TB Diagnostics

Whole-genome sequencing (WGS) has revolutionized TB diagnostics by enabling rapid and comprehensive identification of M. *tuberculosis* strains, drug resistance mutations, and transmission dynamics.

Applications of WGS in TB

1. **Identification of Drug Resistance Mutations:**
   - WGS enables the detection of resistance-associated mutations in genes such as *rpoB*, *katG*, *gyrA*, and *inhA*.
   - Provides insights into emerging resistance patterns and informs treatment regimens.
2. **Epidemiological Surveillance:**
   - Helps track TB outbreaks and transmission chains in communities.
   - Identifies genomic variations that distinguish different M. *tuberculosis* lineages.
3. **Strain Typing and Phylogenetics:**
   - WGS provides precise strain characterization, aiding in understanding TB evolution and spread.
   - Supports differentiation between reinfection and relapse cases.
4. **Rapid Diagnostics:**
   - Compared to traditional culture-based DST, WGS can predict drug susceptibility in days rather than weeks.
   - Facilitates early initiation of effective treatment.

Challenges in Implementing WGS

- High cost and requirement for sophisticated laboratory infrastructure.
- Need for bioinformatics expertise to analyze sequencing data.
- Limited availability in resource-constrained settings.

37. Artificial Intelligence and Machine Learning in TB Research

Artificial intelligence (AI) and machine learning (ML) have emerged as powerful tools in TB diagnostics, treatment monitoring, and epidemiological studies.

AI Applications in TB Diagnosis

1. **AI-Assisted Chest X-Ray Interpretation:**
   - AI models, such as CAD4TB, analyze CXR images to detect TB-related abnormalities.

    - WHO has endorsed AI-assisted CXR interpretation to improve TB screening, particularly in high-burden settings.
2. **Automated Detection of Drug Resistance:**
    - ML algorithms analyze genetic mutations to predict drug resistance profiles.
    - AI-driven DST models enhance diagnostic accuracy and reduce turnaround time.
3. **TB Case Prediction and Surveillance:**
    - AI models analyze demographic, clinical, and environmental data to predict TB risk factors.
    - Supports proactive case detection and public health interventions.
4. **AI in Treatment Monitoring:**
    - AI-powered mobile applications track medication adherence using facial recognition and pill intake monitoring.
    - Helps healthcare providers ensure compliance with TB treatment regimens.

Limitations of AI in TB Research

- Requires high-quality datasets for training models.
- Ethical concerns regarding data privacy and bias in AI models.
- Limited access to AI-based tools in low-resource regions.

38. Host-Directed Therapy and Immunomodulation

Host-directed therapies (HDTs) aim to enhance the host immune response against *M. tuberculosis* while minimizing bacterial survival and resistance.

Key Approaches in Host-Directed Therapy

1. **Targeting the Host Immune Response:**
    - Modulating cytokine pathways (e.g., TNF-α, IL-10) to enhance anti-TB immunity.
    - Enhancing autophagy to promote bacterial clearance.
2. **Repurposing Existing Drugs:**
    - Metformin and statins have shown potential in improving TB treatment outcomes by modifying host metabolism and inflammation.
    - Non-steroidal anti-inflammatory drugs (NSAIDs) are being investigated for their ability to reduce TB-associated lung damage.
3. **Nanotechnology-Based Immunotherapies:**
    - Nanoparticle drug delivery systems enhance drug bioavailability and target infected cells more effectively.

    - Liposomal formulations of rifampicin improve drug penetration into TB granulomas.
4. **Checkpoint Inhibitors in TB Therapy:**
    - Immunotherapy strategies, including PD-1/PD-L1 blockade, are being explored for their role in enhancing host defense mechanisms.

Challenges in Host-Directed Therapy

- Risk of excessive immune activation leading to tissue damage.
- Need for extensive clinical trials to validate HDT efficacy.
- Potential interactions with existing TB drug regimens.

Conclusion

Advances in WGS, AI-driven diagnostics, host-directed therapies, and innovative treatment strategies hold promise for improving TB management. However, overcoming barriers such as drug resistance, diagnostic accessibility, and socioeconomic challenges remains critical. A multidisciplinary approach integrating novel technologies, strong public health policies, and global collaboration is essential for achieving TB eradication in the future.

SECTION 9

PROGRAMS BY THE INDIAN GOVERNMENT TO ELIMINATE TB

Introduction

Tuberculosis (TB) remains a major public health challenge in India, accounting for a significant proportion of the global TB burden. Recognizing the urgent need for TB elimination, the Indian government has implemented several national programs, guidelines, strategies, and milestones to combat the disease. The National Tuberculosis Elimination Program (NTEP), aligned with the WHO's End TB Strategy, aims to make India TB-free by 2025, five years ahead of the global target of 2030.

39. National Tuberculosis Elimination Program (NTEP)

The National Tuberculosis Elimination Program (NTEP), formerly known as the Revised National Tuberculosis Control Program (RNTCP), is India's flagship initiative for TB control and elimination. It was rebranded in 2020 to reflect the shift from TB control to TB elimination.

Objectives of NTEP

- Achieve a TB-free India by 2025.
- Provide universal access to quality TB care and treatment.
- Detect TB cases early and ensure complete treatment adherence.
- Strengthen TB surveillance and research.
- Promote preventive TB care strategies, including contact tracing and vaccination.

Key Components of NTEP

1. **Early Diagnosis and Treatment**
    - Expansion of molecular diagnostic tools like CBNAAT and Truenat.
    - Implementation of universal drug susceptibility testing (UDST).
    - Free TB diagnostics and treatment at public health facilities.
2. **Drug-Resistant TB Management**
    - Deployment of newer drugs like Bedaquiline and Delamanid.
    - Shorter, all-oral regimens for MDR-TB and XDR-TB patients.
3. **Private Sector Engagement**
    - Public-private mix (PPM) model to involve private healthcare providers.
    - Nikshay Portal for tracking private sector TB cases.
4. **Community Engagement and Awareness**
    - TB Champions program to involve TB survivors in advocacy efforts.
    - Community-led active case finding campaigns.

Guidelines and Policies for TB Control in India

The government has released several guidelines to standardize TB care, including:

1. **National Strategic Plan (NSP) for TB Elimination (2017-2025)**
    - Focus on detecting and treating all TB cases.
    - Integration of TB services with primary healthcare.
    - Use of AI-based screening tools for TB detection.
2. **TB Preventive Treatment (TPT) Guidelines**
    - Introduction of shorter regimens for latent TB treatment.
    - Targeting high-risk groups such as household contacts and immunocompromised individuals.
3. **Programmatic Management of Drug-Resistant TB (PMDT) Guidelines**
    - Comprehensive guidance for MDR-TB and XDR-TB treatment.
    - Introduction of newer, safer TB drugs.
4. **NTEP Diagnostic and Treatment Guidelines**
    - Standardized diagnostic algorithms for pulmonary and extrapulmonary TB.
    - Stepwise approach to TB treatment, including first-line and second-line regimens.
    - Use of digital tools like Nikshay for case monitoring and treatment adherence.

TB Elimination Strategies in India

The Indian government follows a multi-pronged approach to achieve TB elimination, including:

1. Active Case Finding (ACF)

- Door-to-door screening for TB in high-burden areas.
- Use of mobile diagnostic units in rural and tribal regions.

2. Universal Drug Susceptibility Testing (UDST)

- Ensuring every TB patient undergoes drug resistance testing before treatment initiation.

3. Strengthening TB Laboratories

- Expansion of CBNAAT, Truenat, and MGIT culture facilities nationwide.

4. Nutrition Support for TB Patients

- Nikshay Poshan Yojana providing direct benefit transfers (DBT) to TB patients for nutritional support.

Key Schemes and Initiatives for TB Elimination

Nikshay Poshan Yojana

- Financial assistance of ₹500 per month for TB patients to support nutrition.

Nikshay Mitra Initiative

- Encourages individuals, corporates, and NGOs to adopt TB patients and provide nutritional and social support.

Universal TB Care under Ayushman Bharat

- Integration of TB diagnosis and treatment into the Ayushman Bharat Health and Wellness Centers (HWCs).

Private Sector Engagement through PPM

- Financial incentives for private practitioners to notify TB cases.
- Strengthening of referral networks between private and public health facilities.

Milestones in India's Fight Against TB

2012: Introduction of CBNAAT (GeneXpert) for rapid TB diagnosis.

2017: Launch of the National Strategic Plan (NSP) with a TB-free India goal by 2025.

2018: Mandatory TB notification policy introduced for private sector reporting.

2019: Implementation of the Nikshay Poshan Yojana for direct benefit transfers.

2020: Revised NTEP guidelines with shorter MDR-TB treatment regimens.

2021: Launch of Nikshay Mitra Initiative to strengthen community participation.

2022: Expansion of AI-assisted TB screening and molecular diagnostic tools.

2023: Introduction of 3HP regimen for preventive treatment of latent TB.

2025: Target year for TB elimination in India.

Working Towards a TB-Free India

1. Strengthening Health Infrastructure

- Upgrading TB laboratories with advanced molecular diagnostics.
- Training healthcare workers on the latest TB treatment protocols.

2. Expanding Research and Innovation

- Encouraging research into new TB vaccines and diagnostics.
- Promoting genomic surveillance to track TB strains and resistance patterns.

3. Ensuring Universal Health Coverage for TB Patients

- Providing free TB drugs and diagnostics at government facilities.
- Expanding insurance coverage for TB treatment under PMJAY (Pradhan Mantri Jan Arogya Yojana).

4. Community Engagement and Awareness Campaigns

- Mass media campaigns to reduce TB stigma.
- Strengthening school-based TB awareness programs.

Conclusion

India's TB elimination program is one of the most ambitious public health initiatives in the world. By implementing innovative strategies, strengthening healthcare infrastructure, engaging communities, and leveraging technology, India is making significant strides toward achieving its goal of a TB-free nation by 2025. Continued political commitment, research investments, and collaborative efforts with international organizations will be key to sustaining progress and ultimately eliminating TB from India.

Section 10

Challenges in Achieving TB Eradication

Challenges in Achieving TB Eradication

Despite advances in diagnostics, treatment, and prevention, TB eradication remains a major global challenge.

40. Barriers in TB Eradication

1. **Emerging Drug Resistance:**
   - The rise of multidrug-resistant TB (MDR-TB) and extensively drug-resistant TB (XDR-TB) complicates treatment efforts.
   - Requires the development of new drugs and rapid DST methods.
2. **Diagnostic Gaps:**
   - Limited access to rapid and accurate TB diagnostics in low-resource settings.
   - Need for affordable point-of-care testing solutions.
3. **Treatment Adherence Issues:**
   - Lengthy TB treatment regimens lead to poor patient adherence.
   - Novel shorter treatment regimens and digital adherence tools are needed.
4. **TB and HIV Co-Infection:**
   - TB remains the leading cause of death among people living with HIV.
   - Integrated TB/HIV programs are essential for improving patient outcomes.
5. **Socioeconomic and Political Barriers:**
   - Poverty, malnutrition, and lack of healthcare access contribute to TB transmission.
   - Political commitment and sustained funding are crucial for TB control programs.

Future Directions in TB Eradication Efforts

- Expansion of universal health coverage to ensure TB diagnosis and treatment access.
- Investment in next-generation TB vaccines with long-lasting immunity.
- Strengthening public-private partnerships for TB research and drug development.

References & Further Reading

World Health Organization (WHO) Reports & Guidelines

1. World Health Organization. Global Tuberculosis Report. Geneva: WHO; [Latest Edition]. Available from: https://www.who.int/tb/publications/global_report/en/
2. World Health Organization. Guidelines for Treatment of Tuberculosis. Geneva: WHO; [Latest Edition].
3. World Health Organization. Consolidated Guidelines on Tuberculosis. Geneva: WHO; [Latest Edition].
4. World Health Organization. The End TB Strategy. Geneva: WHO; 2015.

Books & Textbooks

5. Bloom BR, ed. Tuberculosis: Pathogenesis, Protection, and Control. Washington, D.C.: ASM Press; 1994.
6. Schlossberg D. Tuberculosis. 7th ed. New York: Springer; 2016.
7. Schaaf HS, Zumla A. Tuberculosis: A Comprehensive Clinical Reference. Elsevier; 2009.
8. Murray PR, Rosenthal KS, Pfaller MA. Medical Microbiology. 9th ed. Elsevier; 2020.

Microscopy & Culture Methods

9. Cattamanchi A, Davis JL, Worodria W, et al. Poor performance of universal sample processing method for diagnosis of pulmonary tuberculosis by smear microscopy and culture. J Clin Microbiol. 2009;47(10):3039-3041.
10. Siddiqi K, Lambert ML, Walley J. Clinical diagnosis of smear-negative pulmonary tuberculosis in low-income countries: The current evidence. Lancet Infect Dis. 2003;3(5):288-296.

Molecular Diagnostics

11. Pai M, Nicol MP, Boehme CC. Tuberculosis diagnostics: State of the art and future directions. Microbiol Spectr. 2016;4(5):10.1128/microbiolspec.TBV-0016-2016.
12. Helb D, Jones M, Story E, et al. Rapid detection of Mycobacterium tuberculosis and rifampin resistance by use of on-demand, near-patient technology. J Clin Microbiol. 2010;48(1):229-237.
13. Dorman SE, Schumacher SG, Alland D, et al. Xpert MTB/RIF Ultra for detection of Mycobacterium tuberculosis and rifampicin resistance: A

prospective multicentre diagnostic accuracy study. Lancet Infect Dis. 2018;18(1):76-84.

Interferon-Gamma Release Assays (IGRAs)

14. Pai M, Zwerling A, Menzies D. Systematic review: T-cell-based assays for the diagnosis of latent tuberculosis infection: An update. Ann Intern Med. 2008;149(3):177-184.
15. Chee CB, Reves R, Zhang Y, Belknap R. Latent tuberculosis infection: Opportunities and challenges. Respirology. 2018;23(10):893-900.

Drug Susceptibility Testing (DST)

16. WHO. Technical Report on Critical Concentrations for Drug Susceptibility Testing of Medicines Used in the Treatment of Drug-Resistant Tuberculosis. Geneva: WHO; 2018.
17. Zhang Y, Yew WW. Mechanisms of drug resistance in Mycobacterium tuberculosis: Update 2015. Int J Tuberc Lung Dis. 2015;19(11):1276-1289.
18. Balabanova Y, Ignatyeva O, Fiebig L, et al. Multidrug-resistant tuberculosis in Russia: Clinical characteristics, analysis of second-line drug resistance, and associated risk factors. Emerg Infect Dis. 2015;21(11):2048-2057.

Radiology & Imaging in TB Diagnosis

19. Pande T, Cohen C, Pai M, et al. Computer-aided detection of pulmonary tuberculosis on digital chest radiographs: A systematic review. Int J Tuberc Lung Dis. 2016;20(9):1226-1230.
20. Hwang EJ, Park S, Jin KN, et al. Development and validation of a deep learning-based automatic detection algorithm for active pulmonary tuberculosis on chest radiographs. Clin Infect Dis. 2019;69(5):739-747.

National Guidelines

21. Centers for Disease Control and Prevention (CDC). Treatment of Tuberculosis, American Thoracic Society, CDC, and the Infectious Diseases Society of America. MMWR Recomm Rep. 2003;52(RR-11):1-77.
22. Indian Revised National TB Control Programme (RNTCP). Guidelines for TB Control in India. Ministry of Health and Family Welfare, Government of India, 2020.

23. European Centre for Disease Prevention and Control (ECDC). European guidance on the management of MDR-TB and XDR-TB. Stockholm: ECDC; 2017.

Advances in TB Research

24. Sharma SK, Mohan A. Multidrug-resistant tuberculosis: A menace that threatens to destabilize tuberculosis control. Clin Chest Med. 2019;40(4):701-720.
25. Wright C, Burgess G, Dunn L, et al. Nanotechnology-based diagnostic tools for tuberculosis. Int J Nanomedicine. 2020;15:7327-7345.
26. Gootenberg JS, Abudayyeh OO, Kellner MJ, et al. Multiplexed and portable nucleic acid detection platform with Cas13, Cas12a, and Csm6. Science. 2018;360(6387):439-444.

www.ingramcontent.com/pod-product-compliance
Ingram Content Group UK Ltd.
Pitfield, Milton Keynes, MK11 3LW, UK
UKHW061550190726
13845UKWH00030B/1099

9 789334 258417